RAPID
INTERPRETATION

OF

EKG's

...a programmed course

by

Dale Dubin, M.D.

First Edition Copyright © 1970 COVER Inc.
  first printing, April, 1970
  second printing, May, 1970
  third printing, July, 1970
  fourth printing, October, 1970

Second Edition Copyright © 1971 COVER Inc.
  fifth printing, February, 1971
  sixth printing, May, 1971
  seventh printing, July, 1971
  eighth printing, November, 1971
  ninth printing, March, 1972
  tenth printing, May, 1972
  eleventh printing, August, 1972
  twelfth printing, November, 1972
  thirteenth printing, April, 1973
  fourteenth printing, December, 1973
  fifteenth printing, June, 1974

Third Edition Copyright © 1974 COVER Inc.
  sixteenth printing, October, 1974
  seventeenth printing, February, 1975
  eighteenth printing, August, 1975
  nineteenth printing, April, 1976
  twentieth printing, December, 1976
  twenty-first printing, July, 1977
  twenty-second printing, January, 1978
  twenty-third printing, October, 1978
  twenty-fourth printing, May, 1979

twenty-fifth printing, February, 1980
twenty-sixth printing, October, 1980
twenty-seventh printing, May, 1981
twenty-eighth printing, February, 1982
twenty-ninth printing, September, 1982
thirtieth printing, June, 1983
thirty-first printing, October, 1983
thirty-second printing, August, 1984
thirty-third printing, October, 1985
thirty-fourth printing, November, 1986
thirty-fifth printing, December, 1987
thirty-sixth printing, April, 1988
thirty-seventh printing, December, 1988

Fourth Edition Copyright © 1989 COVER Inc.
  thirty-eighth printing, February, 1989
  thirty-ninth printing, September, 1989
  fortieth printing, March, 1990
  forty-first printing, December, 1991
  forty-second printing, July, 1993
  forty-third printing, October, 1994

Fifth Edition Copyright © 1996 COVER Inc.
  forty-fourth printing, February, 1996
  forty-fifth printing, November, 1996
  forty-sixth printing, March, 1997
  forty-seventh printing, April 1998
  forty-eighth printing, October 1999

Published by:
COVER Publishing Company
P. O. Box 1092
Tampa, Florida 33601
U.S.A.

Telephones:
In U.S.: 1-800-441-8398
Outside U.S.: 813-238-0266
FAX: 813-238-1819
E-mail: CoverPub@GTE.net

Library of Congress Catalog Card Number 88-072108
ISBN 0-912912-02-2

International Availability of
Rapid Interpretation of EKG's

Rapid Interpretation of EKG's has been the international best seller for over thirty years. It is printed in 27 foreign language editions, which are available through publishers in most major countries, and some smaller countries.

The English edition of *Rapid Interpretation of EKG's*, now updated yearly, is available internationally through the internet. We have three internet sites to provide efficient book fulfillment to any location worldwide. Books can be ordered from any country, using major credit cards. The internet sites provide foreign currency conversion information for instant value determination in all mediums of exchange.

Our internet sites display a brief and interesting presentation about *Rapid Interpretation of EKG's* for each of three medical disciplines:

Web Sites:

Physicians and medical students: **theMDsite.com**

Nurses and nurses in training: **CardiacMonitors.com**

Emergency medical personnel: **EmergencyEKG.com**

about sharing...

My most sincere thanks to those persons, worldwide, who took their personal time to send EKG tracings. I am truly grateful. However, the number of people donating tracings* has grown exponentially, making the publication of their names (as I've done previously) virtually impossible.

All of you will observe both classical and unusual tracings that should be saved (use a copier to obtain EKG's committed to a patient's chart) for your personal collection to be shared intellectually with others. Your peers rely on you to share your very special knowledge.

The spirit of unselfish sharing of your knowledge continues to improve the level of care in this crucial medical discipline.

—DD

*I enthusiastically collect and study 12 lead EKG's, strips of classical and unusual tracings, and even those rolls of "code" tracings that are usually discarded. They may be sent to me via the publisher, COVER, Inc., P.O. Box 1092, Tampa, FL 33601. I regret that I cannot acknowledge all tracings. This rescued trash is an invaluable treasured resource; please know that it is appreciated!

ACKNOWLEDGMENTS

With humility and gratitude,
  I acknowledge my indebtedness:

To God for the inspiration and for my persistent survival in spite
  of deadly warning shots. I do understand.

To all my mentors from whom I have learned principles of
  electrocardiography.

To all my family, living and deceased.

To my computer gurus, George Watson and Paul Heinrich, whose graphic
  artistry and knowledge of computer science made this possible.
  A special thanks to Diane Oliver, whose practical savvy and computer
  graphic expertise made this edition much easier to comprehend.

To Dr. Mikel Rothenberg, Dr. John Desmond, and Kathleen Dubin, J.D.,
  whose professional advice, proofing, and editing are greatly appreciated.

To Mike Allison, R.N. for medical photography.

To Francesca Lala for technical and supratentorial assistance.

And to my publisher, COVER Publishing Company, for their great
  understanding and cooperation. My association with the publisher
  represents the closest possible concert between author and publisher.

Some computer graphic illustrations utilize portions of *LifeART* clip art.

DEDICATION

To those from whom I have learned:

Dr. Paul Dudley White
Dr. George C. Griffith
Dr. Willard J. Zinn
Dr. Henry J. L. Marriott
Dr. Charles Fisch
Dr. William L. Martz
Dr. Nathan Marcus
Dr. Richard G. Connar
Dr. Jose Dominguez
Dr. Louis Cimino
Dr. David Baumann
Dr. Suzanne Knoeble
Dr. Dale Dubin

TABLE OF CONTENTS

"To make a great dream come true, the first requirement is a great capacity to dream; the second is persistence – a faith in the dream."

Hans Selye, M.D.

Before You Begin . . .

First read each caption and associate it with the graphic illustration.

    Master each illustration.

Then carefully read the programmed text, filling in each blank as you go.

- If you have to return to the illustration to refresh your memory—that's even better—. . . because each time you review an illustration, the visual image will be more indelibly impressed in your memory.
- Programmed instruction is intellectual growth by graduated increments of related concepts.

    . . . and it works because it is really an exciting audience participation course, and you are the audience.

"Lasting knowledge results from understanding."

Happy Learning,

Dale Dubin

Dale Dubin, M.D.

Most teachers are knowledgable.
Good teachers are intelligent.
Great teachers are patient.
Exceptional teachers are students themselves.

          D.D.

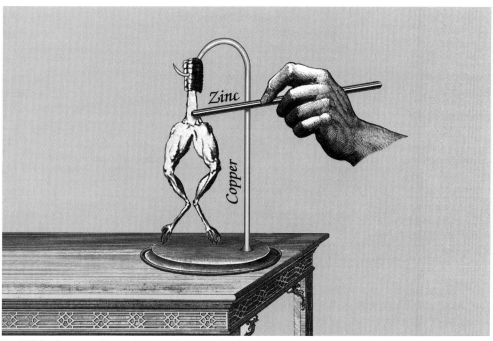

In 1790, the usually sedate audience of scientists gasped in disbelief as Luigi Galvani, with a flare of showmanship, made a dead frog's legs dance by electrical stimulation.

Galvani knew that completing a circuit connecting dissimilar metals
to the legs of a recently deceased frog would create a stimulating
_____ current.   electrical

The resulting electrical current would stimulate the frog's legs
to jump, and with repeated stimuli he could make them _____.   dance

NOTE: But in those times, bringing a dead frog "back to life"
was a shocking and ghastly "supernatural" feat.
(And Galvani loved it!)*

*Get yourself a warm cup of coffee, relax and enjoy...the rest is just as easy and entertaining.

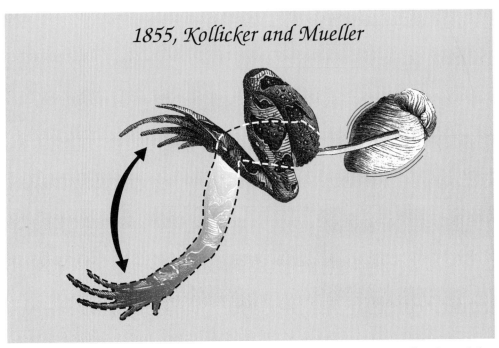

1855, Kollicker and Mueller

While conducting basic research around 1855, Kollicker and Mueller found that when a motor nerve to a frog's leg was laid over its isolated beating heart, the leg kicked with each heartbeat.

"Eureka!" they thought, "the same electrical stimulus that causes a frog's leg to kick must cause the heart to _____."

beat

So it was logical for them to assume that the beating of the heart must be due to a rhythmic discharge of _____ stimuli.

electrical

NOTE: And thus an association between the rhythmic pumping of the heart and electrical phenomena was scientifically established. Very basic and very important.

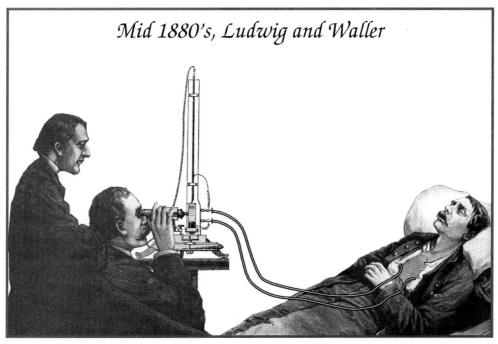

Mid 1880's, Ludwig and Waller

In the mid 1880's, while using a "capillary electrometer", Ludwig and Waller discovered that the heart's rhythmic electrical stimuli could be monitored from a person's skin.

This apparatus consisted of sensor electrodes, which were placed on a man's _____ and connected to a Lippman capillary electrometer, which used a capillary tube in an electric field to detect faint electrical activity.
skin

The level of fluid in the capillary tube moved with the rhythm of the subject's _____-beat...very interesting.
heart

This apparatus was a little too unsophisticated for clinical application, or even for economic exploitation, but it was _____ interesting.
very

NOTE: This momentous achievement opened the door for recording the electrical activity of the heart from (intact) skin surfaces.

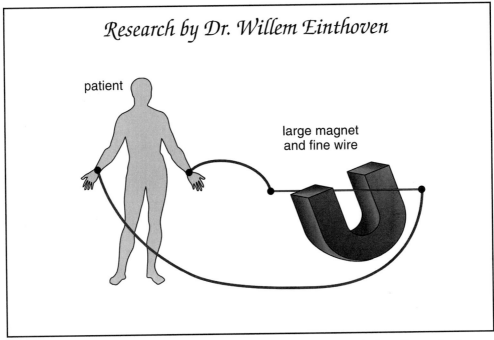

Research by Dr. Willem Einthoven

patient

large magnet
and fine wire

Enter Willem Einthoven, a brilliant scientist who suspended a silvered wire between the poles of a magnet.

Two skin sensors (electrodes) placed on a man were then connected across the silvered wire, which ran between the two poles of the _____.

magnet

The silvered _____ (suspended in the magnetic field) twitched to the rhythm of the subject's heartbeat.

wire

This was also very interesting, but _____ wanted a timed record.

Einthoven

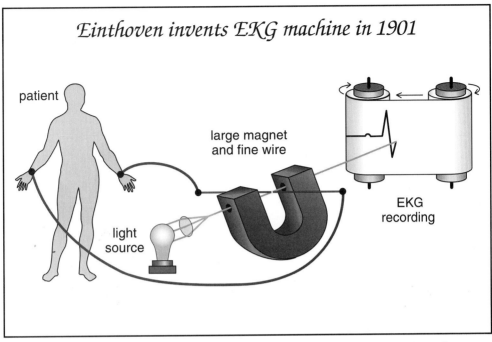

Einthoven invents EKG machine in 1901

patient

large magnet
and fine wire

light
source

EKG
recording

So Einthoven projected a tiny light beam through holes in the magnet's poles, across the twitching silvered wire. The wire's rhythmic movements were recorded as *waves* (named P, QRS, and T) on a moving scroll of photographic paper.

Very clever, that Einthoven! The _____ rhythmic
movements of the wire (representing the heartbeat) created
a bouncing shadow…

…that was recorded as a _____ series of rhythmic
distinct waves in repeating cycles.

He named the waves of each cycle (alphabetically)
P, QRS, and ____. T

NOTE: "Now," thought the clever Einthoven, "we can record
a heart's *abnormal* electrical activity…and compare it to the
normal." And thus a great diagnostic tool, his "<u>e</u>lectro<u>k</u>ardio<u>g</u>ram"
evolved around 1901. Let's see how it works...

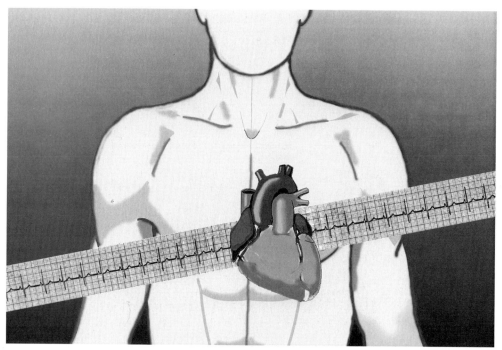

The *electrocardiogram* (EKG) records the electrical activity of the heart, providing a record of cardiac electrical activity, as well as valuable information about the heart's function and structure.

The electrocardiogram is known by the three letters _____,   EKG
and it provides us with a record of cardiac electrical activity and
valuable information about the heart's function and structure.

NOTE: Since the time of Einthoven's "<u>e</u>lectro<u>k</u>ardiogram," the medical profession has used the letters EKG to represent the electrocardiogram. Some say that "ECG" is more correct, and you may see it used in some texts. However, Medicine honors tradition, and EKG has been used for years. Also, ECG sounds like EEG (the brain wave recording), and this can cause misunderstanding and confusion.

The EKG is inscribed on a ruled paper strip that gives
us a permanent _____ of cardiac activity and the   record
health status of the heart. Cardiac monitors and cardiac
telemetry provide the same information.

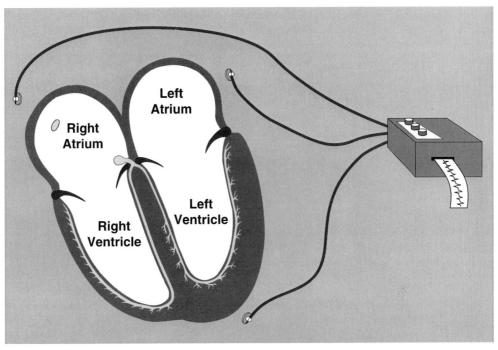

The electrocardiogram records the electrical impulses that stimulate the heart muscle ("myocardium") to contract.

The information recorded on the EKG represents the
_____ impulses from the heart.   electrical

Most of the information on the EKG represents electrical
impulses that _____ the heart to contract.   stimulate

NOTE: The EKG also yields valuable information about the
heart's resting and recovery phases.

When the myocardium (*cardium* = heart, *myo* = muscle)
is electrically stimulated, it _____.   contracts

NOTE: This illustration is intended to familiarize you with the
simplified cross-section of the heart. The chambers are identified,
and you should know them, for this drawing will be used often.

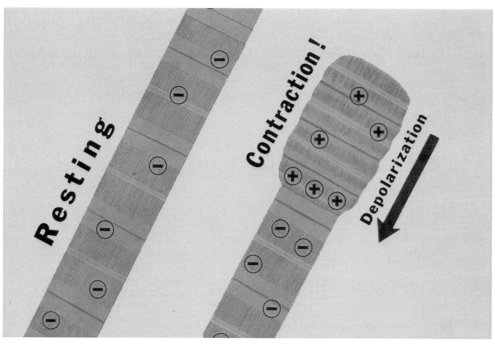

When at rest, the muscle cells of the heart have negatively charged ("polarized")
interiors, but when they are "depolarized" by an electrical stimulus, they contract.

While in the resting state, the cells of the heart are *polarized*,
the inside of every cell being _____ charged at rest.   negatively

NOTE: In the strictest sense, a resting, polarized cell has a
negatively charged interior and a positively charged outside surface,
but for simplicity we will consider only the negative interior.

The interiors of the myocardial cells, which are usually
negatively charged, become _____-ly charged,   positive
stimulating the cells to contract.

The electrical stimulation of the heart's muscle cells* that
makes them _____ is called "depolarization."   contract
Depolarization moves as a wave through the myocardium.

* Just as the heart muscle is called the myocardium, its cells are called "myocytes".

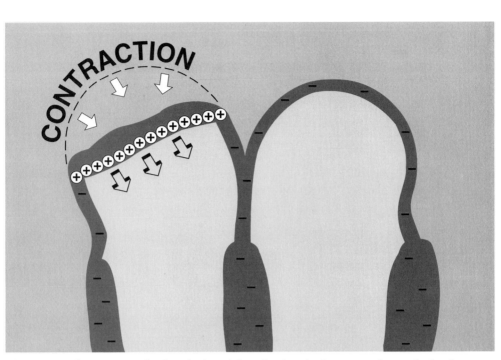

A progressive wave of stimulation (*depolarization*) passes through the heart, causing contraction of the myocardium.

Depolarization may be considered an advancing wave
of _____ charges within the myocardium.   positive

   NOTE: The depolarization wave stimulates the myocardial
cells (myocytes) to contract as the charge within each cell
changes to positive.

The electrical stimulus of depolarization causes progressive
contraction of the myocytes, as the wave of _____ charges   positive
advances through the interiors of the cells.

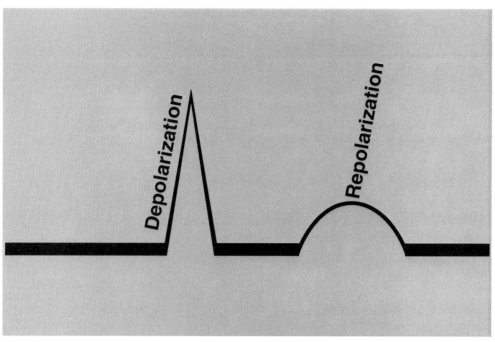

The wave of depolarization (cell interiors become positive), and a phase of *repolarization* (cell interiors return to negative) that follows, are recorded on the EKG as shown.

The stimulating wave of depolarization makes the interiors
of the myocardial cells _____ and stimulates them   positive
to contract.

But then the myocytes regain their resting negative
charge within each of the cells during the phase of
_____ that follows.   repolarization

   NOTE: Repolarization is an electrical phenomenon that, in reality,
   begins immediately after depolarization. The broad hump which we
   see on EKG is really the most active phase of repolarization.

Myocardial stimulation by _____ is   depolarization
recorded on the EKG as shown above. The "recovery" phase
that follows is known as _____.   repolarization
(See illustration.)

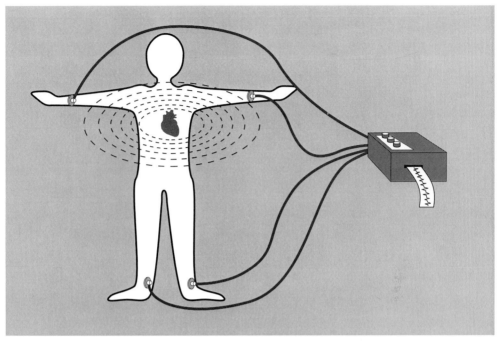

Sensors called "electrodes" are placed on the skin to detect this electrical activity as it passes through the heart. The EKG machine records this activity on paper as an electrocardiogram.

Both depolarization and repolarization are
_____ phenomena.   electrical

The electrical activity of the heart may be detected and recorded from the _____ surface by sensitive monitoring equipment, including EKG machines, cardiac monitors, and telemetry devices.   skin

The EKG records the electrical activity of the heart using skin sensors called _____.   electrodes

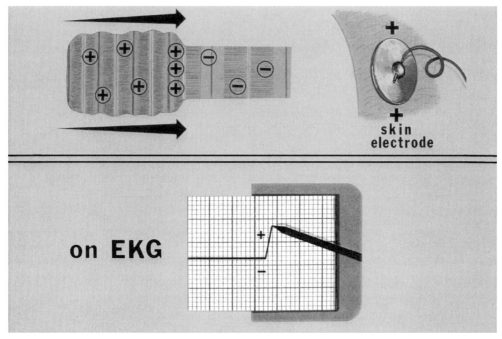

As the positive wave of depolarization within the heart cells advances toward a positive electrode, there is a positive (upward) deflection recorded on EKG.

NOTE: "Positive electrode," of course, refers to a positive electrode actively recording a patient's EKG.

An advancing wave of depolarization may be considered a moving wave of _____ charges.   positive

When this wave of positive charges moves toward a positive _____ electrode, there is a simultaneous upward deflection recorded on EKG.   skin

When you see an upward wave on EKG, you know that it represents a depolarization wave moving toward a _____ electrode.   positive

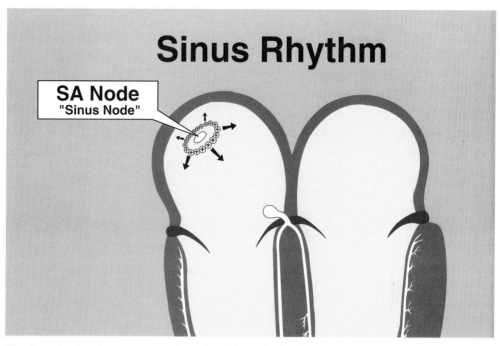

The heart's dominant pacemaker, the *SA Node,* begins the impulse of depolarization which spreads outward in wave fashion, stimulating the atria to contract.

NOTE: The SA Node ("Sinus Node") is the heart's dominant pacemaker, and its pacing activity is known as a "Sinus Rhythm." The ability to generate pacemaking stimuli is known as **automaticity**. Other focal areas of the heart that have automaticity are called "*automaticity foci*".

The SA Node, located in the upper-posterior wall of the right
_____, initiates a depolarization stimulus at regular intervals   atrium
to accomplish its pacemaking responsibility.

Each depolarization wave (of + charges) proceeds outward
from the SA Node and stimulates both atria to _____.   contract

The ability of the SA Node to generate pacemaking stimuli
is known as _____.   automaticity

NOTE: The depolarization stimulus proceeds away from the
SA Node in all directions. Imagine the atria as a pool of water.
A pebble dropped in at the SA Node produces an enlarging,
circular wave (depolarization) that spreads outward from it. Atrial
depolarization is a spreading wave of positive charges within the atrial
myocardial cells. Let's read this page again.

13

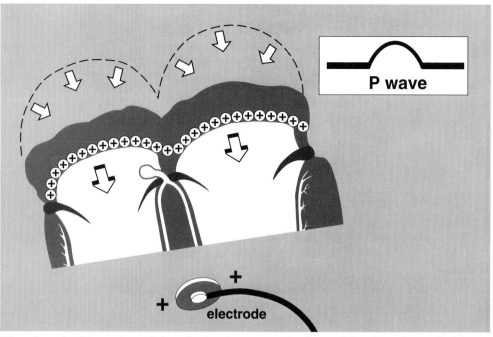

The electrical impulse of depolarization spreads through both atria, and this produces a *P wave* on the EKG.

NOTE: The illustration depicts the positive wave of atrial depolarization advancing toward a positive electrode, producing an upward (positive) P wave on EKG.

The wave of depolarization sweeping through the atria can be detected by sensitive _____ electrodes.

skin

Atrial depolarization is recorded as a ___ wave on EKG.

P

So when we see a P wave on an electrocardiogram, we know that it represents atrial _____, electrically speaking.

depolarization (stimulation)

NOTE: The atria also have a specialized conduction system, which we will examine later (page 97, if you're curious).

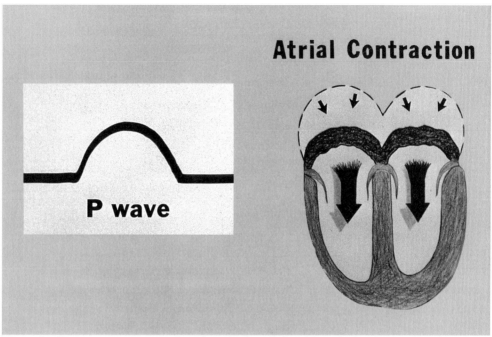

Thus the P wave represents the electrical activity (depolarization) of both atria, and it also represents the simultaneous contraction of the atria.

As the wave of depolarization passes through both atria, there is a simultaneous wave of atrial _____.   contraction

So the P wave represents the depolarization and contraction of both _____.   atria

NOTE: In reality, contraction of the atria lasts longer than the duration of the P wave. However, we'll still consider that a P wave = atrial contraction. This simultaneous contraction of the atria forces the blood they contain to pass through the Atrio-Ventricular (AV) valves between the atria and the ventricles.

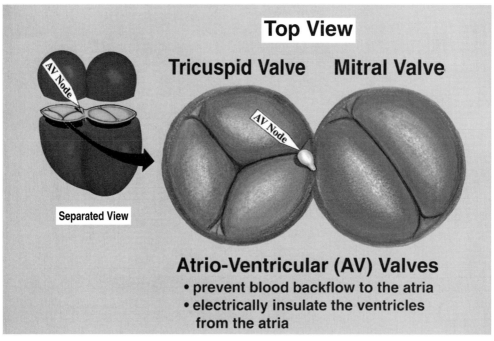

Top View

Tricuspid Valve   **Mitral Valve**

AV Node

AV Node

Separated View

Atrio-Ventricular (AV) Valves
• prevent blood backflow to the atria
• electrically insulate the ventricles
from the atria

The *Atrio-Ventricular (AV) valves* prevent ventricle-to-atrium blood backflow, and electrically insulate the ventricles from the atria...except for the *AV Node*.

When the ventricles contract, the blood they contain cannot
flow back to the atria due to the very efficient _____ valves.   AV

The *mitral* and *tricuspid (AV) valves* lie between the atria
and the ventricles, thereby acting to electrically _____   insulate
the ventricles from the atria...

...leaving only the _____ Node as the sole pathway to conduct   AV
the depolarization stimulus (from the atria) through the fibrous
AV valves to the ventricles.

NOTE: The AV Node is just above, but continuous with a specialized
conduction system that distributes depolarization to the ventricles very
effectively. Now let's do a quickie review of the mechanical pumping
processes that move blood through the chambers of the heart.

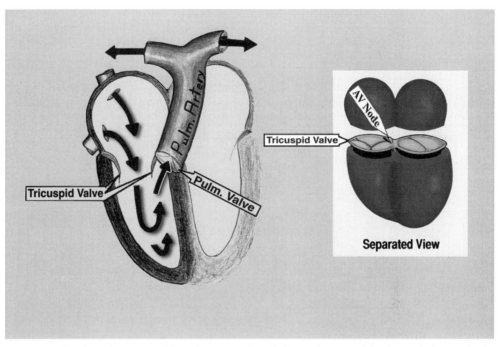

Separated View

Oxygen-depleted venous blood enters the right atrium and is forced through the tricuspid valve into the right ventricle, which forces it into the lungs.

NOTE: Tricuspid is right side.

The right side of the heart (right atrium and right ventricle) receives under-oxygenated venous blood from all over the body, and pumps it into the _____.

lungs

The right ventricle contracts, forcing the under-oxygenated venous blood through the *pulmonary valve* into the _____ *artery* and thence to the lungs.

pulmonary

NOTE: Remember, both atria contract simultaneously, and both ventricles contract together also. However, the right and left sides of the heart have different responsibilities.

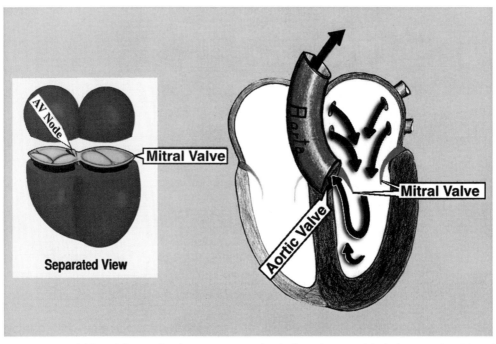

Oxygenated blood from the lungs enters the left atrium, which forces the blood through the mitral valve into the left ventricle, which in turn pumps it into the *aorta*.

NOTE: Mitral is left side.

The left atrium contracts, forcing oxygenated blood through the
_____ valve into the left ventricle.   mitral

Then the muscular left ventricle contracts, forcing oxygenated blood
through the *aortic valve* into the _____. (That's too easy!)   aorta

Both atria contract simultaneously, then both _____   ventricles
contract simultaneously.

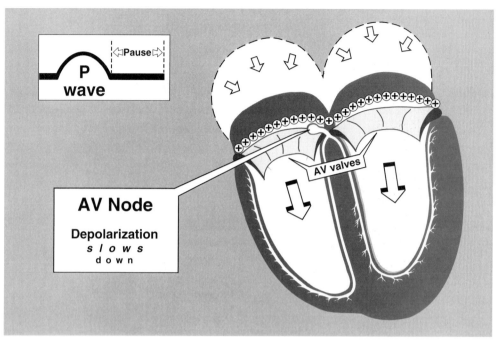

The atrial depolarization stimulus reaches the AV Node, where depolarization s l o w s, producing a brief pause, thus allowing the blood in the atria to enter the ventricles.

NOTE: Of course you remember that the AV Node is the only electrical conduction pathway between the atria and the ventricles.

Because the stimulus of depolarization slows within the AV Node, there is a brief delay or _____ before depolarization can pass into the ventricles.

pause

This brief pause allows the blood from the atria to pass through the AV valves and into the _____.

ventricles

NOTE: At this point, we are correlating electrical activity with mechanical physiology. The atria contract, forcing blood through the AV valves, but it takes a little time for the blood to flow through the valves into the ventricles (hence the necessary pause that produces a short piece of flat baseline after each P wave on the EKG). Please review the illustration again.

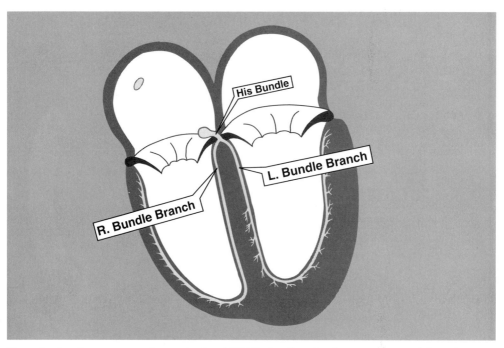

Depolarization passes through the AV Node slowly, but upon reaching the *ventricular conduction system,* depolarization conducts very rapidly through the *His Bundle* and the *Left* and *Right Bundle Branches* and their subdivisions.

Although this stimulus is retarded in its passage through the
AV Node, depolarization conducts rapidly through the
ventricular conduction system beginning at the _____ Bundle.   His

Depolarization passes slowly through the AV Node,
then rapidly down the His Bundle to the Right and Left
_____ Branches.   Bundle

After this stimulus has rapidly passed through the His Bundle
and the Bundle Branches and their subdivisions, depolarization
is quickly distributed to the myocardial cells (*myocytes*) of
the _____.   ventricles

NOTE: The ventricular conduction system originates at the His Bundle,
which penetrates the AV valves, then it reaches the interventricular septum,
where it immediately divides into the Right and Left Bundle Branches. The
His *Bundle* and both *Bundle* Branches are "bundles" of rapidly conducting
*Purkinje fibers**, that's why depolarization passes quickly through them.

*Texts in the past (including this one) have INCORRECTLY implied that only the terminal filaments were
   Purkinje fibers. Study NOTE and learn it correctly.

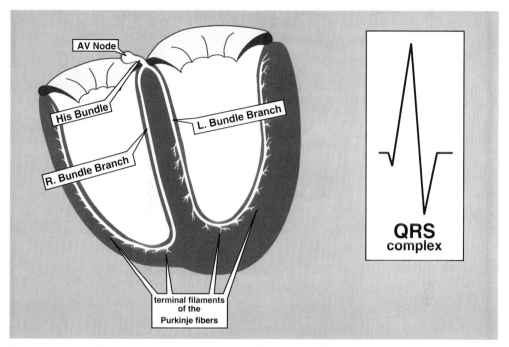

The terminal filaments of the Purkinje fibers distribute the depolarization stimulus to the ventricular myocardial cells. Depolarization of the ventricular myocardium produces a *QRS complex* on EKG.

NOTE: The ventricular conduction system is composed of bundles of rapidly-conducting Purkinje fibers that conduct depolarization at high speed away from the AV Node. The Purkinje fibers terminate in tiny filaments that depolarize the myocardial cells of the ventricles. The (rapid) passage of depolarization down the ventricular conducting system is too weak to record on EKG; however, depolarization of the ventricular myocardium records as the QRS complex.

The depolarization stimulus progresses slowly through the AV Node, then it conducts rapidly through the His Bundle to the Right and Left Bundle Branches into the terminal filaments of the Purkinje fibers that depolarize the _____ myocardial cells.   ventricular

NOTE: The terminal filaments of the Purkinje fibers spread out just beneath the *endocardium* that lines both ventricular cavities, so ventricular depolarization begins at the lining and proceeds toward the outside surface (*epicardium*) of the ventricles. The Purkinje fibers branch and subdivide at the endocardial lining, but they really do not penetrate into the myocardium. Since that's almost impossible to depict in a two-dimensional drawing, please recognize the limits of the illustration and remember it correctly.

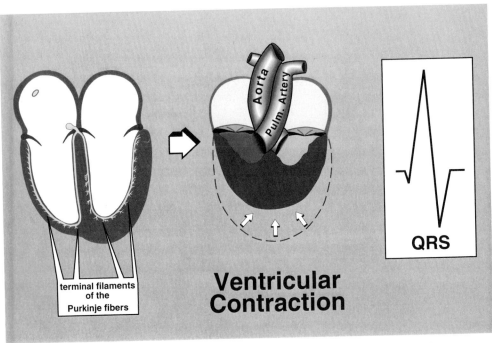

terminal filaments
of the
Purkinje fibers

**Ventricular
Contraction**

QRS

The entire ventricular conduction system consists of rapidly conducting
Purkinje fibers. The terminal filaments of the Purkinje fibers depolarize the
ventricular myocardium, initiating ventricular contraction while inscribing a
QRS complex on EKG.

The terminal filaments of the Purkinje fibers rapidly conduct
the depolarization _____ to the myocardial cells that lie   stimulus
just beneath the endocardial lining of both ventricles.

NOTE: Remember that the entire ventricular conduction system, i.e., the His
Bundle through the terminal filaments, is composed of Purkinje fibers.

Depolarization of the ventricular myocytes (myocardial cells)
produces a ____ complex on the electrocardiogram and   QRS
initiates contraction of the ventricles.

NOTE: The QRS complex actually represents the beginning of ventricular
contraction. The physical event of ventricular contraction actually lasts longer
than the QRS complex, but we will still consider the QRS complex as generally
representing the occurrence of ventricular contraction. So the QRS complex is
an electrocardiographic recording of ventricular depolarization, which causes
ventricular contraction. Still with me?

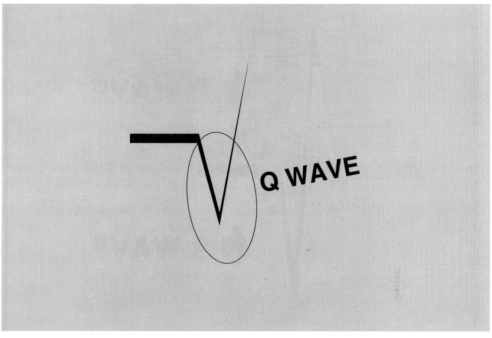

The *Q wave* is the first downward stroke of the QRS complex, and it is followed by an upward *R wave*. The Q wave is often not present.

The Q wave*, when present, always occurs at the
_____ of the QRS complex and is   beginning
the first downward deflection of the complex.

The downward Q wave is followed by an upward ____   R
wave.

NOTE: If there is any upward deflection in a QRS complex that appears before a "Q" wave, it is not a Q wave, for by convention, when present, the Q wave is always the first wave in the complex.

_____

* It is now popular to use small (non-capital) letters to designate small waves in the QRS complex, for instance a "q" (small, lower case q) wave is a small wave.

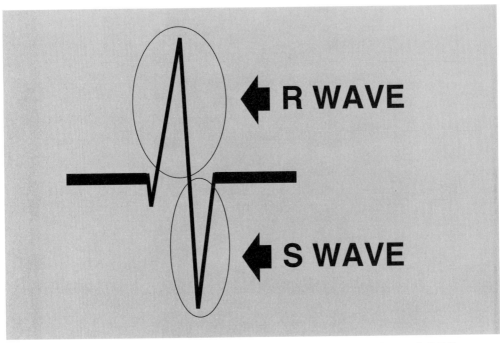

The upward R wave is followed by a downward *S wave*. This total QRS complex represents the electrical activity of ventricular depolarization.

The first upward deflection of the QRS complex is the
_____.

R wave

Any downward stroke PRECEDED by an upward stroke is an _____.

S wave

The complete QRS complex can be said to represent _____ depolarization (and the initiation of ventricular contraction).

ventricular

NOTE: The upward deflection is always called an R wave. Distinguishing between the downward Q and S waves really depends on whether the downward wave occurs before or after the R wave. The Q occurs before the R wave, and the S wave follows the R. Just remember your alphabet.

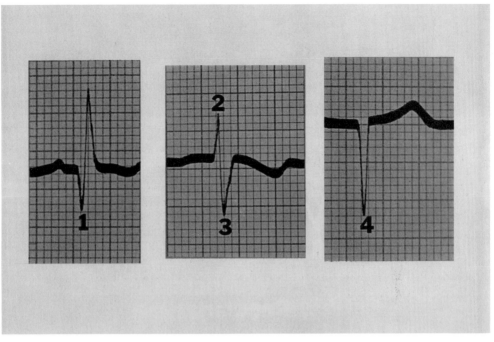

Name each of the numbered waves.

1. _____   Q wave

2. _____   R wave

3. _____   S wave

4. _____   QS wave

NOTE: Number 4 is a little unfair. Because there is no
upward wave, we cannot determine whether number 4 is a
Q wave or an S wave. Therefore it is called a *QS wave*,
and it is considered to be a Q wave when we look for Q's.

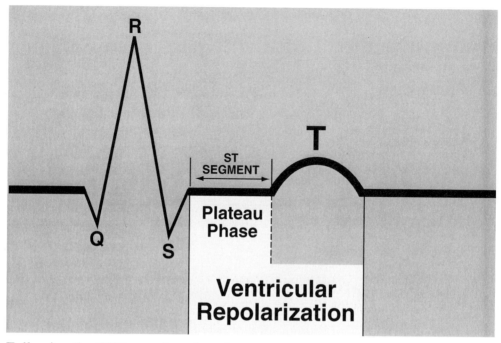

Following the QRS complex, there is a segment of horizontal baseline known as the *ST segment*, and then a broad *T wave* appears.

The horizontal segment of baseline that follows
the QRS complex is known as the _____ segment.   ST

After the QRS there is a segment of horizontal baseline,
followed by a broad hump known as the _____ wave.   T

NOTE: The ST segment is horizontal, flat, and most importantly,
it is normally level with other areas of the baseline. If the ST segment
is elevated or depressed beyond the normal baseline level,
this is often an important sign of serious pathology that may
indicate immanent problems.

NOTE: The ST segment represents the "plateau" (initial) phase
of ventricular repolarization. Ventricular repolarization
is rather minimal during the ST segment.

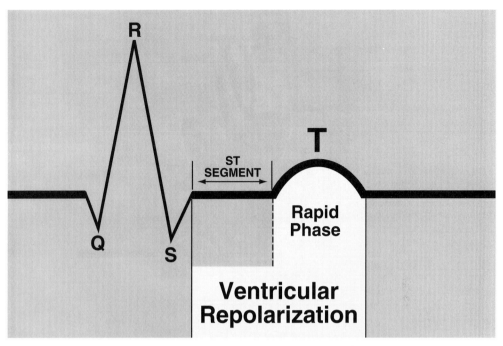

The T wave represents the final, "rapid" phase of ventricular repolarization, during which ventricular repolarization occurs quickly and effectively.

Repolarization occurs so that the ventricular myocardial cells can recover their resting negative charge within each _____, and then they can be depolarized again.

cell
(myocyte)

Even though the T wave is usually a low, broad hump, it represents the _____ phase of ventricular repolarization.

rapid

Repolarization of the ventricular myocytes begins immediately after the QRS and persists until the end of the _____ wave.

T

NOTE: Ventricular *systole** (contraction) begins with the QRS and persists until the end of the T wave. So ventricular contraction (systole) spans depolarization and repolarization of the ventricles. This is a convenient physiological marker.

* Pronounced "SISS-toe-lee"

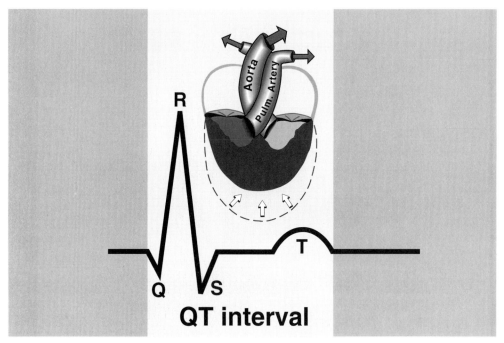

QT interval

Since ventricular systole lasts from the beginning of the QRS until the end of the T wave, the *QT interval* has clinical significance.

The QT interval represents the duration of ventricular
_____ and is measured from the beginning of the   systole
QRS until the end of the T wave.

NOTE: Since repolarization comprises most the QT interval, some say that it is a good indicator of repolarization. Long QT intervals often warn that a patient is vulnerable to rapid ventricular rhythms.

NOTE: With rapid heart rates both depolarization and repolarization occur faster for greater efficiency, so the QT interval varies with rate. Precise QT interval measurements are corrected for rate, and they're called QTc values. As a simple rule of thumb, the QT interval is considered normal when it is less than half of the R-to-R interval at normal rates.

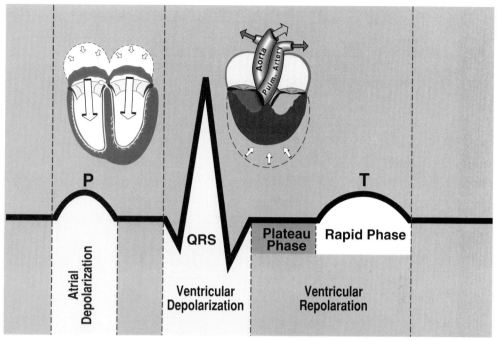

A *cardiac cycle* is represented by the P wave, the QRS complex, the T wave, and the baseline that follows until another P wave appears. This cycle is repeated continuously. Please study the illustration to make certain that you understand every event in sequence.

NOTE: Physiologically, a cardiac cycle represents atrial systole (atrial contraction), followed by ventricular systole (ventricular contraction), and the resting stage that follows until another cycle begins.

Atrial depolarization (and contraction) is represented by the ___ wave.   P

Ventricular depolarization (and contraction) is represented by the _____ complex.   QRS

NOTE: In reality, atrial contraction lasts longer than the P wave, and ventricular contraction lasts longer than the QRS complex, but you already knew that.

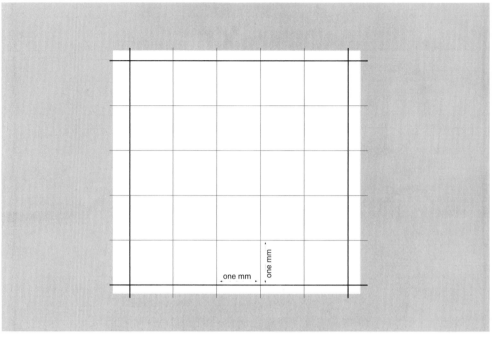

The EKG is recorded on ruled (graph) paper. The smallest divisions are one millimeter (mm) squares.

The EKG is recorded on a long strip of _____   ruled
paper, although some EKG machines record many   (graph)
different leads simultaneously on a large sheet.

The smallest divisions are one _____   millimeter
long and one _____ high.   millimeter

Between the **heavy** black lines there are ___ small squares.   5
Each large square is formed by **heavy** black lines on each side,
and each side is five mm long.

NOTE: As with all graphs, the time axis is horizontal and moves left to right,
like we read. So timed events on EKG are measured left to right and similarly,
cardiac monitors display a time axis which reads from left to right.

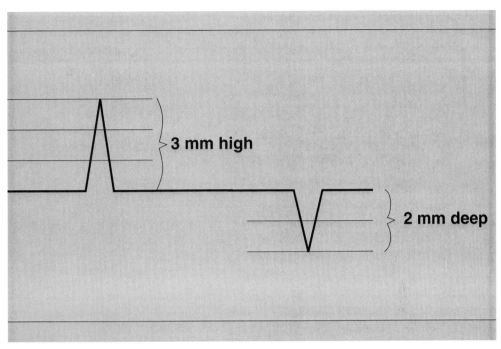

The height and depth of a wave are measured vertically in millimeters, and this represents a measure of voltage*.

The height or depth of waves is measured
in _____ and is a measure of voltage.   millimeters

NOTE: The *deflection* of a wave is the <u>direction</u> in which it records on EKG; for instance, the "upward deflection" or "downward deflection" of a wave. However, the *amplitude* of a wave is the <u>amount</u> (in millimeters) of upward deflection or downward deflection. The height or depth of a wave (i.e., its amplitude) is a measure of voltage

The first wave in the illustration has an upward deflection of
3mm in _____.   amplitude

NOTE: The elevation or depression of segments of baseline is also measured vertically in millimeters, just as we measure waves.

* Ten millimeters vertically represents one millivolt (mV), however, in practice, one usually speaks of "millimeters" of height or depth (waves) and the same for elevation or depression of baseline segments.

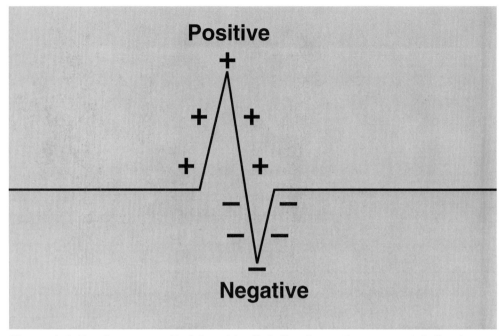

Upward deflections are called "positive" deflections. Downward deflections are called "negative" deflections.

Positive deflections are _____ on the EKG.   upward

Negative deflections are _____ on the EKG.   downward

NOTE: When a wave of stimulation (depolarization) advances toward a positive skin electrode, this produces a positive (upward) deflection on EKG. You will recall that depolarization is an advancing wave of positive charges within the cardiac myocytes. So with depolarization, the advancing wave of positive intracellular charges produces a positive deflection on EKG as this wave moves toward a positive electrode. Be positive!

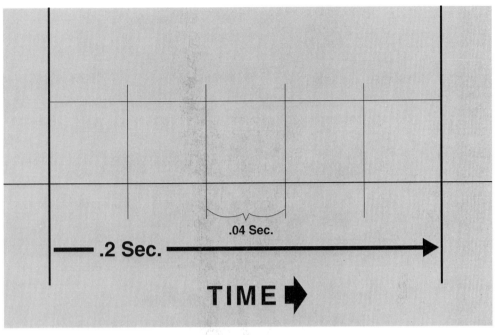

The horizontal axis represents time.

Between the **heavy** black lines there are __ small squares.   5

The amount of time represented by the distance between
two **heavy** black lines is _____.   .2 of a second
                                                                    (2/10 of a second)

Each small division (measured horizontally between
two fine lines) represents _____.   .04 of a second
                                                                    (that's four
                                                                    hundredths!)

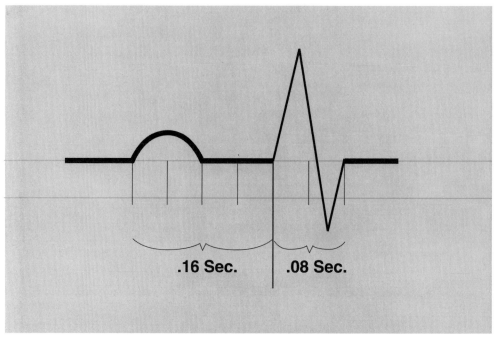

By measuring along the horizontal axis, we can determine the duration of any part of the cardiac cycle.

The duration of any wave may be determined by measuring along the horizontal _____.

axis

,

Four of the small squares represents _____ of a second.

.16
(sixteen hundredths)

The amount of EKG graph paper that passes out of the EKG machine in .12 second is _____ small squares. (You don't have to be a mathematician to read EKG's.)

three
(3)

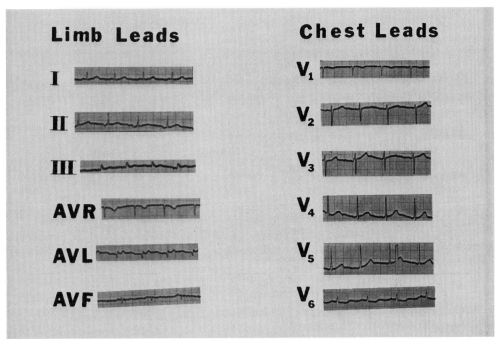

The standard EKG is composed of 12 separate *leads**.

A standard EKG is composed of six _____ leads, recorded by using arm and leg electrodes and...   limb

...there are also six _____ leads obtained by placing a suction cup electrode at six different positions on the chest.   chest

NOTE: Leads not considered "standard" may be monitored from various locations on the body as needed for special diagnostic requirements.

* Rhymes with seeds.

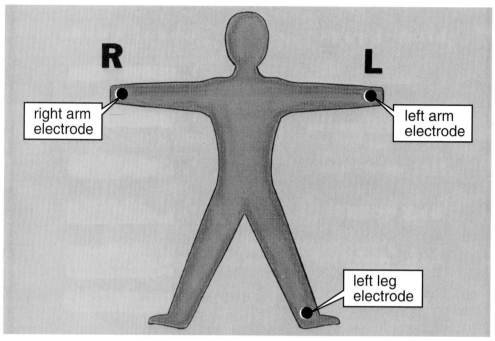

To obtain the *limb leads*, electrodes are placed on the right arm, the left arm, and the left leg.

By placing electrodes on the right and left arms and the left leg, we can obtain and record the _____ leads.

limb

NOTE: The electrocardiogram is still recorded using these three limb locations for the electrodes.

The placement of these _____ is the same as originally used by Willem Einthoven.

electrodes

NOTE: Two electrodes are used to record a lead. A different pair is used for each lead.

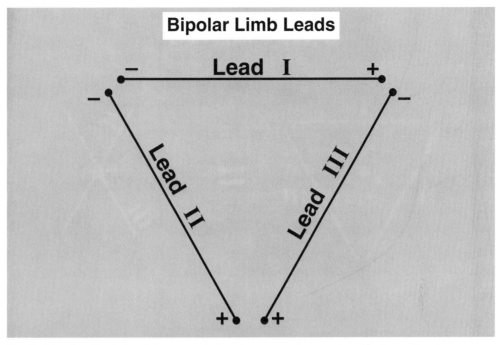

Each *bipolar* limb lead is recorded using two electrodes. So by selecting a different pair of electrodes for each lead, we create three separate bipolar limb leads (*lead I*, *lead II*, and *lead III*) for recording.

Each limb lead consists of a pair of electrodes, one is positive and one is _____, so these   negative
leads are called "bipolar" limb leads.

Lead I is horizontal, and its left arm electrode is _____,   positive
while its right arm electrode is negative.

When we consider lead III, the left arm electrode is now _____, and the left leg electrode is   negative
positive.

NOTE: The engineering wonders of the EKG machine permit us to make any skin electrode positive or negative depending on which pair of electrodes (that is, which lead) the machine is recording.

NOTE: The bipolar limb lead configuration is sometimes called "Einthoven's triangle."

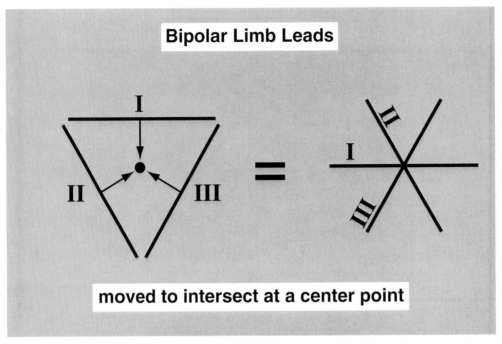

Bipolar Limb Leads

moved to intersect at a center point

By pushing the three (bipolar) limb leads to the center of the triangle, we produce three intersecting lines of reference.

The triangle has a center, and each _____ may be moved   lead
to that center point.

By pushing leads I, II, and III to the center of the
triangle, three intersecting lines of _____ are formed.   reference

Although the three bipolar limb leads may be moved to
the _____ of the triangle, they remain at the same angles   center
relative to each another. (They're still the same leads, yielding the
same information.)

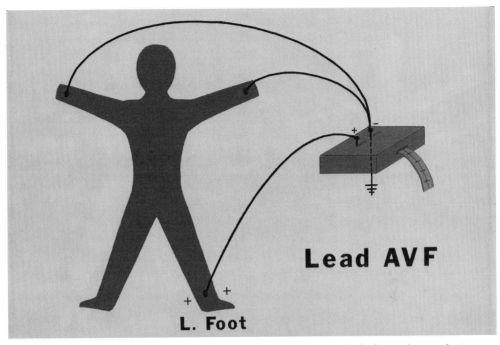

Lead AVF

L. Foot

Another lead is the *AVF* lead. The AVF lead uses the left foot electrode as positive and both arm electrodes as a common ground (negative). Let's ignore the right foot for now.

The AVF lead uses the left foot electrode as _____.   positive

In AVF both the right and left arm electrodes are
channeled into a common ground that has a
_____ charge.   negative

NOTE: Dr. Emanuel Goldberger, who designed and introduced the "Augmented" limb leads, discovered that in order to record a lead in this manner, he had to amplify (Augment) the Voltage in the EKG machine to get a tracing of the same magnitude as leads I, II, and III. He named this lead: A (Augmented), V (Voltage), F (left Foot), and he went on to produce two more leads using this same technique.

ASIDE: Your deductive mind tells you that lead AVF is a mixture of leads II and III...just what Dr. Goldberger was trying to accomplish! Therefore lead AVF is a cross between (and oriented between) those two bipolar limb leads. Now, let's create two more augmented leads.

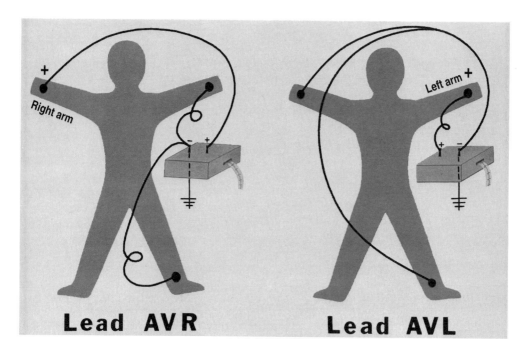

Lead **AVR**   Lead **AVL**

The remaining two augmented limb leads, *AVR* and *AVL*, are obtained in a similar manner (still ignoring the right foot sensor).

For the AVR lead the <u>R</u>ight arm electrode is positive, and the remaining two electrodes are _____.   negative

To obtain the AVL lead, the <u>L</u>eft arm electrode is made _____; the other two electrodes are negative.   positive

NOTE: Although the right foot has an electrode connected to the EKG machine, it is not functional when recording the augmented leads.

NOTE: AV<u>R</u> — Right arm positive
        AV<u>L</u> — Left arm positive
        AV<u>F</u> — Foot (left foot) positive
(These augmented limb leads are sometimes called the "unipolar" limb leads, stressing the importance of the positive electrode.)

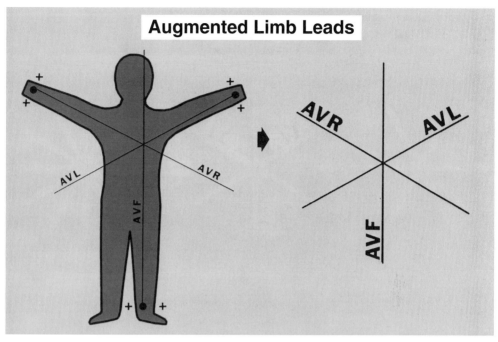

Augmented Limb Leads

The augmented limb leads, AVR, AVL, and AVF, intersect at different angles (than those produced by the bipolar limb leads) and produce three other intersecting lines of reference.

AVR, AVL, and AVF are the augmented (or "unipolar")
_____ leads.   limb

These augmented limb leads _____ at   intersect
60 degree angles, but the angles differ from those
formed by bipolar limb leads, I, II, and III.

Leads AVR, AVL, and AVF intersect at angles _____   different
from leads I, II, and III.   In fact, leads AVR, AVL, and AVF
split the angles formed by leads I, II, and III.

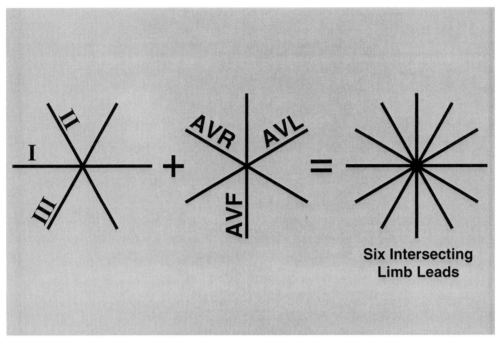

Six Intersecting Limb Leads

All six limb leads (I, II, III, and AVR, AVL, and AVF) meet to form six intersecting reference lines that lie in a flat plane on the patient's chest.

The six limb leads are the three bipolar limb leads, I, II, III, and the three augmented limb leads, _____, _____, and _____.

AVR , AVL
AVF

If the intersecting bipolar limb leads I, II, and III are superimposed on augmented limb leads AVR, AVL, and AVF, we have ___ neatly intersecting leads (one every 30 degrees).

6

These six limb leads may be visualized as lying in a flat plane over the patient's _____.

chest

NOTE: The flat plane of the limb leads is called the *frontal plane*, in case anyone asks you.

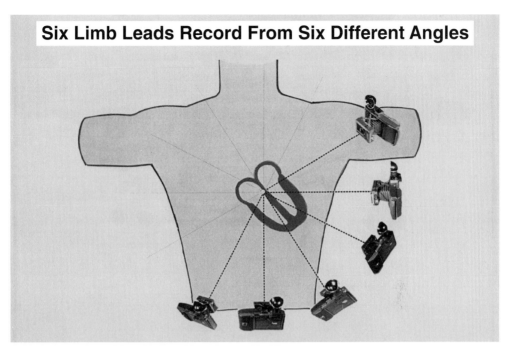

Six Limb Leads Record From Six Different Angles

Each lead records from a different angle (viewpoint), thus each limb lead (I, II, III, AVR, AVL, and AVF) provides a different view of the same cardiac activity.

The EKG records the same cardiac _____ in   activity each lead.

The waves look different in various leads because the heart's electrical activity is recorded from a different _____   angle for each lead.   (viewpoint)

NOTE: Remember that the heart's electrical activity never changes from lead to lead, but the electrode positions are different for each lead. So the tracing looks slightly different in each lead, as the angle from which we record the electrical activity changes from lead to lead. Remember, a wave of depolarization is a progressive wave of POSITIVE charges passing through the myocardial cells. So, if a depolarization wave moves toward a POSITIVE electrode, this produces a POSITIVE (upward) deflection on the EKG (or monitor) for that particular lead. (A little repetitious, but it is *so* important!)

43

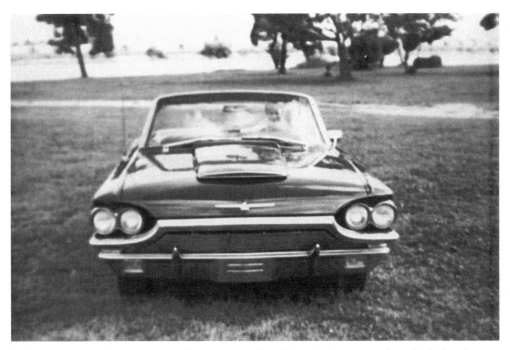

It is conceptually necessary for you to visualize the intersecting limb leads. Why? Can you identify this car?

NOTE: This page sure seems empty, doesn't it?

NOTE: Automobile experts are encouraged not to recognize the car for the sake of understanding the analogy.

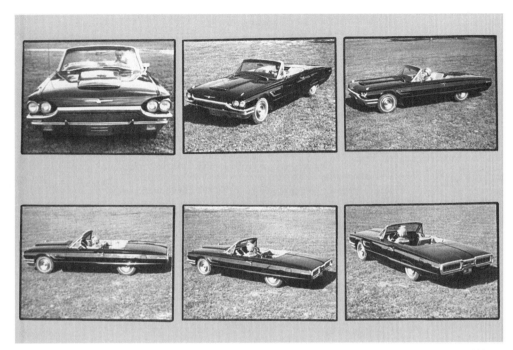

If you observe this same object from six different reference points, you will recognize the car.

NOTE: You can't see the car's back bumper in the photo at top left. But with progressively different views you can determine more about the bumper (or even the driver). Similarly, it may be difficult to see a specific wave in a given lead, but with six different lead positions, it is certain to show up better in other leads.

NOTE: Observation from six different angles is better than one. Thus recording cardiac electrical activity from six different angles gives us a much greater and more accurate perspective. At this point you can take a sip of coffee and relax. The car probably has been recycled into new objects by now, but the concept should always remain in your mind.

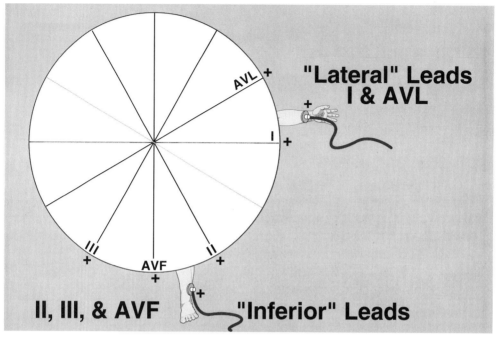

The importance of the positive electrode is emphasized by the practical grouping of limb leads according to the location of the positive electrode for each lead.

Leads I and AVL are called the "lateral leads" (left lateral understood) because each has a _____ electrode positioned laterally on the left arm.

positive

Leads II, III, and AVF are called the "inferior leads" because each of these leads has a positive electrode positioned inferiorly on the left _____.

foot

NOTE: So now we can easily identify depolarization toward (or even away from) the patient's left side, and the same for depolarization directed inferiorly toward (or even away from) the left foot. The "inferior leads" and the "lateral leads" include 5 of the 6 limb leads. These are not arbitrary designations. These terms are common cardiology parlance and have important clinical/diagnostic significance. Know and understand them.

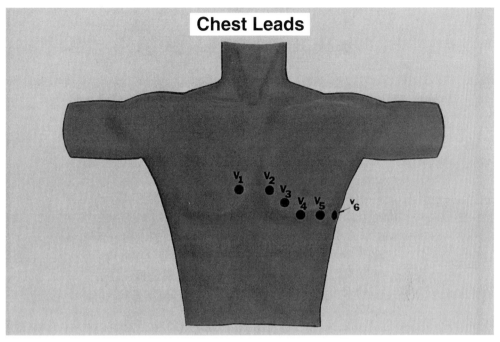

Chest Leads

To obtain the six standard *chest leads,* a positive electrode (suction cup) is placed at six different positions (one for each lead) on the chest.

The six chest leads are recorded from six progressively different positions around the _____. (See illustration.)   chest

For each of the chest leads, the suction cup electrode that is placed on the chest is considered _____.   positive

The chest leads are numbered from V_1 to V_6 and are positioned in successive steps from the patient's right to his or her left side. Notice how the chest leads cover the _____ in its normal   heart anatomical position within the chest.

NOTE: Traditionally a suction cup electrode records the chest leads, however adhesive metal electrodes are now commonly used. Because the electrode for the chest leads is always POSITIVE, a depolarization wave moving toward a given chest electrode produces a POSITIVE (upward) deflection in that chest lead of the EKG tracing.

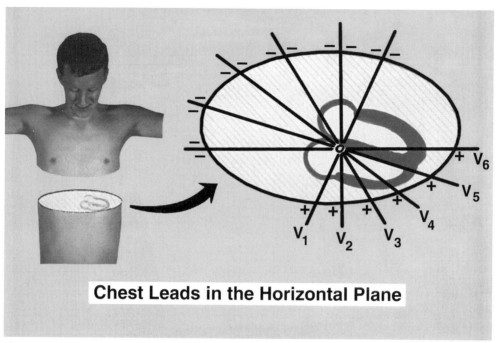

Chest Leads in the Horizontal Plane

Each of the chest leads* is oriented through the AV node and exits through the patient's back, which is negative.

NOTE: The plane of the chest leads (called the *horizontal plane*) cuts the body into top and bottom halves.

The electrode for each of the chest leads is always considered _____ (positive or negative).

positive

If leads V_1 through V_6 are imagined to be the spokes of a wheel, the center of the wheel is the _____.

AV Node

Lead V_2 describes a straight line directly from the front to the back of the patient. In lead V_2 the patient's back is considered _____ (positive or negative).

negative

* The chest leads (also called the "precordial" leads) were introduced by Dr. Frank Wilson.

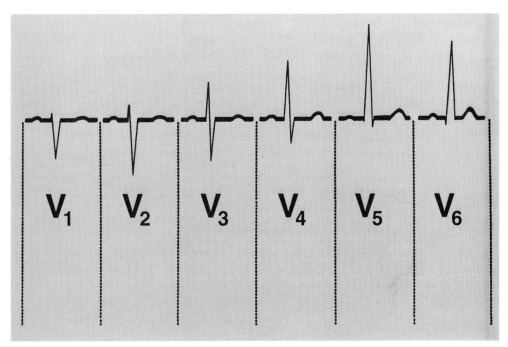

By examining an EKG, you will notice that the waves of the six chest leads show progressive changes from V_1 to V_6.

NOTE: When observing the chest leads from V_1 to V_6 you will see gradual changes in all the waves (as the electrode position changes for each successive lead).

Considering the V_1 chest lead, the QRS complex is mainly
_____ (positive or negative) normally.   negative

In chest lead V_6 the QRS complex is usually mainly
_____ (positive or negative).   positive

So considering the V_6 chest lead, we know that the positive wave
of ventricular depolarization (represented by the QRS complex)
is moving _____ the POSITIVE chest electrode of V_6 toward
(if you don't understand this well, take another look at page 12).

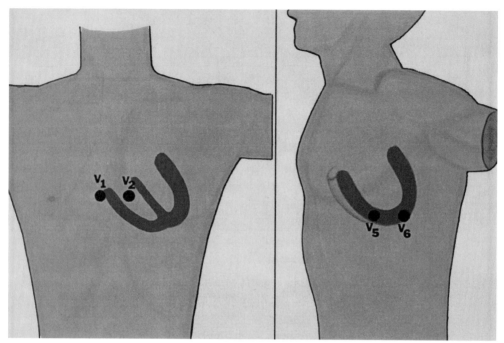

Leads V_1 and V_2 are oriented over the right side of the heart, while V_5 and V_6 are oriented over the left side of the heart. (See Below)

Leads V_1 and V_2 are called the "_____" chest leads.

right

The two chest leads oriented over the left side of the heart are ___ and ___, (and are called the "left" chest leads).

V_5 and V_6

A depolarization wave moving toward the (positive) chest electrode in lead V_6 causes an _____ deflection on the EKG tracing of this lead. (NOW you understand!)

upward (positive)

• Acls Book says Vi and V2 face the septum of the heart

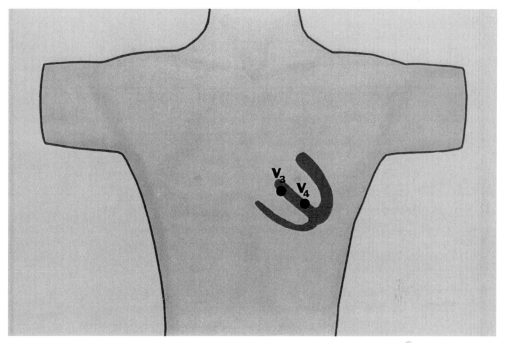

Leads V₃ and V₄ are oriented over the *interventricular septum.* (See Below)

Leads V₃ and V₄ are oriented over the area of the
interventricular _____.

septum

NOTE: The interventricular septum is a common wall shared
by the right and left ventricles, so this septum separates the
cavity of the right ventricle from the cavity of the left ventricle.
The Right and the Left Bundle Branches course through the
interventricular septum.

• ACLS Book says V3, V4 face the Anterior chest wall
   (Anterior wall of left ventricle)

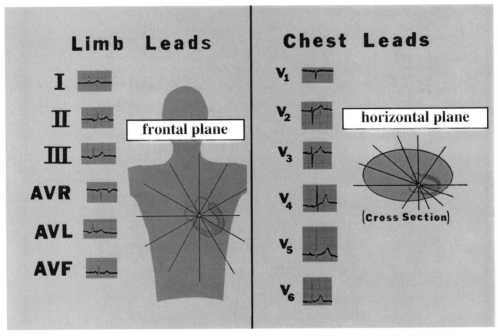

On the standard EKG tracing there are six chest leads and six limb leads. This is the 12 lead electrocardiogram.

The six limb leads all lie in the _____ plane, which can be visualized over the patient's chest.

frontal

The six chest leads lie in the horizontal plane and are arranged in progressive order from V_1 to ____.

V_6

The six chest leads are recorded using a positive electrode which is placed at six specific anatomical positions on the chest encircling the heart in the _____ plane.

horizontal

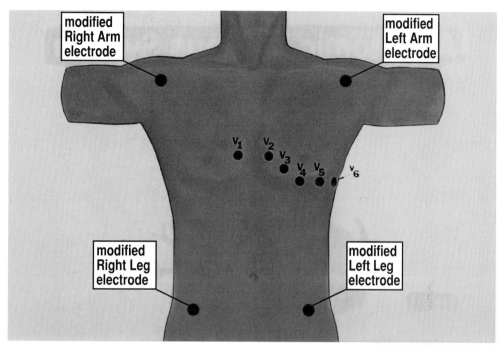

The six limb leads also can be recorded by using carefully positioned electrodes on the trunk of the patient. The special electrode placement (above) used for exercise ("stress") testing can be used to record each of the twelve EKG leads.

NOTE: An EKG recorded from a carefully positioned trunk electrode can record the same information (same accuracy and same amplitude) as an ankle or wrist electrode for a given limb lead. Precise accuracy of electrode placement on the trunk* is essential, however.

Cardiac monitoring in hospital rooms, as well as in the emergency department, surgery, recovery room, coronary care, and intensive care, is carried out using carefully positioned electrodes on the patient's _____ to monitor classical limb (and other) leads.

trunk

Paramedics and many Emergency Medical Technicians use trunk* _____ for diagnostic purposes and also for telemetry transmission.

electrodes

Now we're ready to tackle the autonomic nervous system...O.K.?

*These are "trunk" but not truly "chest" electrodes, for they often use the shoulders and abdomen as electrode locations. A variety of modifications are commonly used to monitor patients in various settings and circumstances (see page 322).

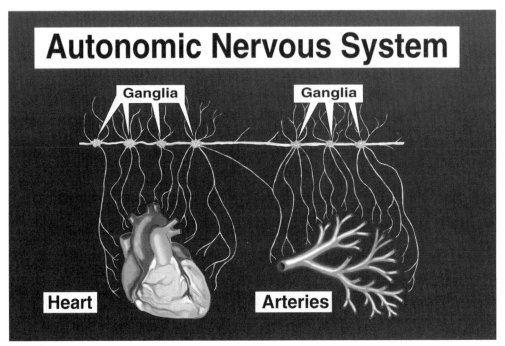

Autonomic Nervous System

Ganglia

Ganglia

Heart

Arteries

The Autonomic Nervous System (ANS) modulates vital functions of all organs by both central nervous system and reflex control, but <u>not</u> by conscious control.

Although the ANS controls all organs and organ systems,
our main concern here is autonomic control of the _____,   heart
and also of the systemic arteries as they relate to blood pressure.

NOTE: The ANS has two divisions that seem difficult to comprehend because one division may stimulate one organ, yet inhibit another organ. Fear not! Think of each division as an electrical system that controls terminal switches called "receptors". In each division, some receptors can stimulate, while its receptors in another area can inhibit. We just need to identify the location of the receptors and what they do at that site. Trust me.

NOTE: Any stimulus originating in the ANS initially passes to a *ganglion**
of nerve cells (cell bodies) for processing, then those cells secondarily
relay the stimulus to the terminal nerve ends. The terminal end of the nerve
fiber is modified into a wide disc, the *synaptic bouton* (bouton is French for
button), which covers receptors on a cell of the organ under ANS control.

* "Ganglion" is singular, "ganglia" is plural.

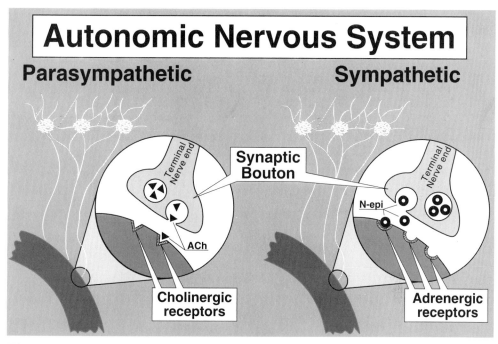

Autonomic Nervous System

Parasympathetic　　　　　　　**Sympathetic**

Terminal Nerve end

Synaptic Bouton

N-epi

ACh

Cholinergic receptors　　　　　　　**Adrenergic receptors**

The ANS consists of a *sympathetic* system and an opposing *parasympathetic* system. Each of these two systems secretes its own *neurotransmitter* from its terminal synaptic boutons in order to activate specific cell receptors.

The terminal <u>sympathetic</u> nerve ends (synaptic boutons) secrete Nor-epinephrine* (N-epi), an <u>adrenaline</u>-like neurotransmitter that activates specific _____ receptors called *adrenergic* receptors.　　　cell

NOTE: In the heart, the sympathetic and parasympathetic nervous systems not only have opposite functions, but also opposing effects, that is, they exercise some control of one another.

The terminal <u>parasympathetic</u> nerve ends (synaptic boutons) secrete the neurotransmitter Acetyl<u>choline</u> (ACh), which exclusively activates cell _____ called *cholinergic* receptors.　　　receptors

*Nor-epinephrine, hyphenated for recognition purposes, will be "Norepinephrine" from now on.

Sympathetic Beta (Adrenergic) Receptors
B_1 adrenergic receptors

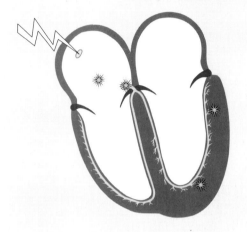

Cardiac Excitatory Effects

⇧ rate of SA Node pacing

⇧ rate of conduction

⇧ force of contraction

⇧ irritability of foci

The heart is stimulated by the sympathetic system through its terminal synaptic boutons, which secrete N-epi onto the β_1 (adrenergic) receptors to elicit an EXCITATORY response.

Norepinephrine, the terminal neurotransmitter of the sympathetic system, stimulates β_1 (adrenergic) receptors, which increase the force of myocardial contraction, and also increase the speed of conduction through the AV Node and the specialized conduction systems of the atria and ventricles, and through the myocardium itself. N-epi also:

...stimulates the SA Node to pace _____,   faster

...increases irritability of atrial and Junctional (page 119)
automaticity _____ and minimally effects ventricular foci.   foci

This means there are β_1 _____ in, and   receptors*
sympathetic innervation to, all of the above areas.

   NOTE: N-epi's brother, *epinephrine* (also called "adrenaline") is secreted into the blood by the adrenal glands. Epinephrine is an even *more potent* stimulator of the heart's β_1 receptors.

* "β_1 adrenergic receptors" is often shortened to "β_1 receptors", but *adrenergic* is understood.

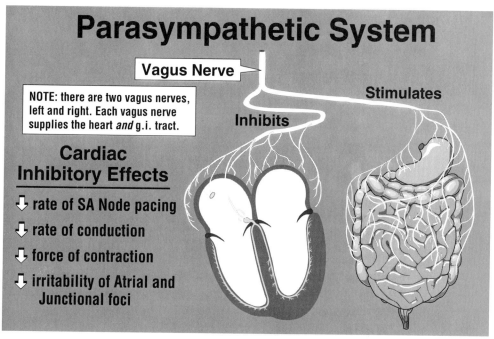

Parasympathetic System

Vagus Nerve

NOTE: there are two vagus nerves, left and right. Each vagus nerve supplies the heart *and* g.i. tract.

Stimulates

Inhibits

Cardiac Inhibitory Effects

⬇ rate of SA Node pacing

⬇ rate of conduction

⬇ force of contraction

⬇ irritability of Atrial and Junctional foci

Parasympathetic nerves release the neurotransmitter acetylcholine (ACh), which activates cardiac cholinergic receptors (most are within the atria) to produce a cardiac INHIBITORY effect. Conversely, the gastrointestinal tract is stimulated by its parasympathetic innervation.

NOTE: The *vagus* nerves are the body's main parasympathetic pathway, so "vagal" stimulation means parasympathetic stimulation, with the understanding that vagal "stimulation" of the heart is inhibitory.

Parasympathetic activation of cholinergic receptors by ACh:
...inhibits the SA Node, decreasing the heart _____;   rate

...depresses irritability of automaticity _____, particularly   foci
  those in the atria and AV Junction;

...diminishes the force of myocardial _____;   contraction

...and decreases the speed of conduction, particularly in
  the AV _____.   Node

NOTE: Despite the parasympathetic system's inhibiting effect on the heart, parasympathetic activation of cholinergic receptors stimulates the gastrointestinal tract. Recalling the agony of severe vomiting or an episode of painful, crampy diarrhea will help you remember the effect of excessive parasympathetic stimulation of the stomach and the bowel.

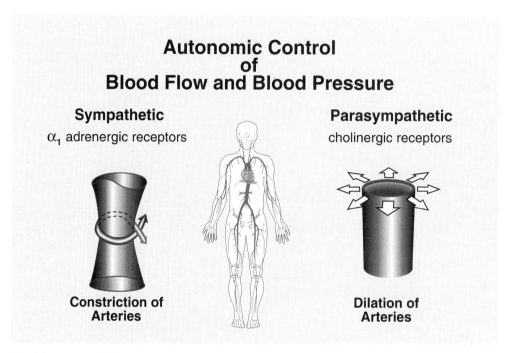

Autonomic Control
of
Blood Flow and Blood Pressure

Sympathetic

α₁ adrenergic receptors

Parasympathetic

cholinergic receptors

Constriction of Arteries

Dilation of Arteries

Besides controlling the SA Node's pacing rate, the Autonomic Nervous System regulates blood flow and blood pressure by modulating arterial constriction and dilation throughout the body.

Sympathetic stimulation of arterial α_1 (adrenergic) receptors constricts arteries throughout the _____, increasing blood   body pressure and blood flow. The α_1 receptors are more responsive to the neurotransmitter N-epi than to circulating epinephrine.

NOTE: By pulling both ends of the Greek *alpha*, the center loop of the letter "α" constricts the artery (see arrows on the α in the illustration). Now you will always remember alpha adrenergic sympathetic effects on systemic arteries.

Parasympathetic activation of arterial (cholinergic) receptors dilates the same arteries as above, reducing blood _____   pressure and blood flow. Not only is there a direct cholinergic inhibitory effect on the arteries, but also there is an inhibitory parasympathetic effect on the sympathetic ganglia that send fibers to the vessels.

NOTE: Blood flow is also very dependent on the heart rate: sympathetic stimulation increases the SA Node pacing rate, while parasympathetic decreases it. Autonomic modulation of the heart rate and systemic blood pressure involves a delicately controlled (parasympathetic—sympathetic) balance to maintain circulatory *homeostasis* (the ideal status quo).

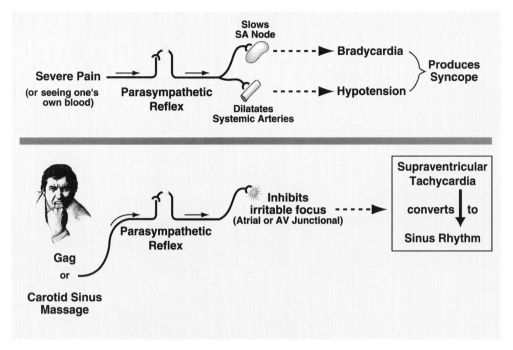

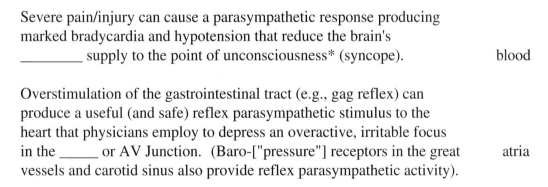

Cardiovascular sensors provide ("afferent") input for parasympathetic reflex mechanisms. These mechanisms delicately counterbalance sympathetic effects to provide physiological homeostasis. Vagal reflexes can produce undesirable symptoms, but can also provide beneficial diagnostic and therapeutic maneuvers.

Severe pain/injury can cause a parasympathetic response producing marked bradycardia and hypotension that reduce the brain's _____ supply to the point of unconsciousness* (syncope).   blood

Overstimulation of the gastrointestinal tract (e.g., gag reflex) can produce a useful (and safe) reflex parasympathetic stimulus to the heart that physicians employ to depress an overactive, irritable focus in the _____ or AV Junction. (Baro-["pressure"] receptors in the great   atria vessels and carotid sinus also provide reflex parasympathetic activity).

NOTE: In normal individuals, pooling of blood in the lower extremities from prolonged standing is compensated by a sympathetic reflex increase in blood pressure and heart rate. In some elderly patients, pooling is excessive and incompletely compensated, so the partially filled ventricles contract rigorously, stimulating parasympathetic mechanoreceptors in the ventricles. This initiates a parasympathetic reflex response to slow the SA Node and further reduce blood pressure. The resulting loss of consciousness is *neuro-cardiogenic syncope.*

*This and other types of vagally mediated syncope are sometimes called "vaso-vagal syncope." Syncope is pronounced "SINK-oh-pee."

> # 1. Rate
>
> # 2. Rhythm
>
> # 3. Axis
>
> # 4. Hypertrophy
>
> # 5. Infarction

Your grasp of the basics and understanding of the autonomic nervous system, will help you to master these five general areas in order to properly interpret an EKG.

The interpretation of an _____ requires consideration of *Rate, Rhythm,*   EKG
Axis, Hypertrophy, and *Infarction.* They are all equally important.

NOTE: Take a moment and examine page 310. This simple methodology is to become your routine. Prepare ahead. <u>Before</u> you begin a chapter, preview its summary (pages 311 to 321), so as you assimilate each chapter, a delightful "aha" will light up your brain as your <u>understanding</u> evolves. This is the foundation of your <u>knowledge</u>.

Ready?

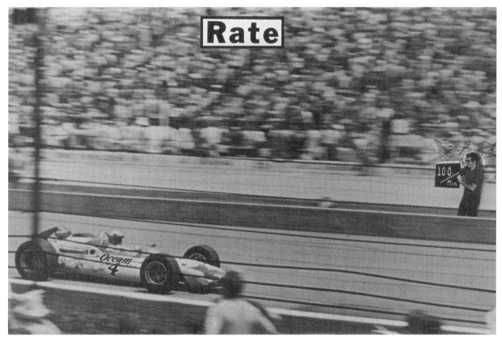

When reading an EKG, you should first consider the rate.

NOTE: The sign in this picture is not informing the driver*
about the rate of his race car. The man holding the sign is
a physician who has been monitoring the driver's transmitted
EKG. The sign is telling the driver about his current
heart rate (he's a little excited).

When examining an EKG, you should determine the
_____ first.   rate

The rate is read as cycles per _____.   minute

Now let's examine where and how the normal heart rate originates..

*With a sincere dedication to Billy Occam, now deceased, who made simplicity a virtue of
  science.

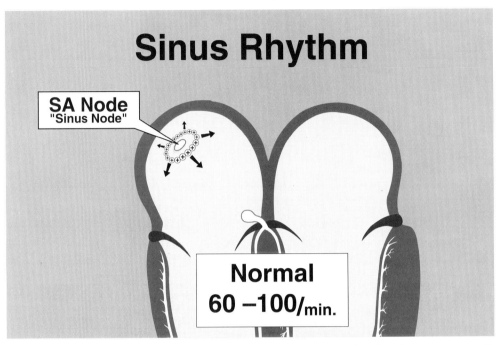

The SA Node (Sinus Node), the heart's pacemaker and the dominant center of automaticity, generates a *Sinus Rhythm*. The SA Node paces at a resting rate range of 60 to 100 per minute.

The heart's normal pacemaker, the _____, generates a continuous series of regular, pacemaking stimuli (this is its "automaticity").

SA Node

The SA Node is located within the upper-posterior wall of the right _____. The SA Node emits a regular series of pacemaking (depolarization) stimuli.

atrium

NOTE: The Sinus Node (SA Node) is the heart's dominant center of automaticity, and the normal, regular rhythm that it generates is called the Sinus Rhythm.

At rest, the Sinus Rhythm maintains a rate of 60 to _____ beats per minute, which is the normal range of the rate of pacing.

100

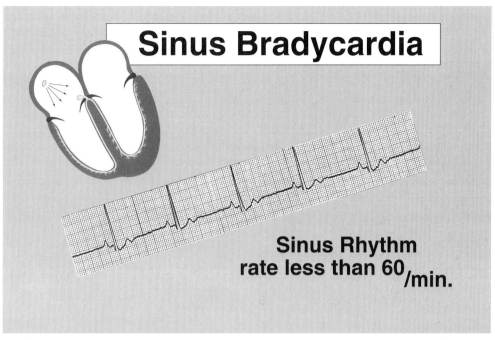

When the Sinus Node (SA Node) paces the heart at a rate slower than 60 per minute, this is called *Sinus Bradycardia.*

   NOTE: "Brady" = slow; "cardia" = heart.

A rhythm originating in the heart's normal pacemaker, the SA Node, with a rate slower than 60 per minute is called Sinus _____. Bradycardia

   NOTE: Sinus Bradycardia is most often caused by parasympathetic excess. Sometimes the slowed heart rate may slow circulation enough to significantly reduce blood flow to the brain and cause *syncope* (loss of consciousness).

Sinus Bradycardia is present if a heart rate of less than one beat per _____ is produced by the Sinus Node.
   second
   (careful!)

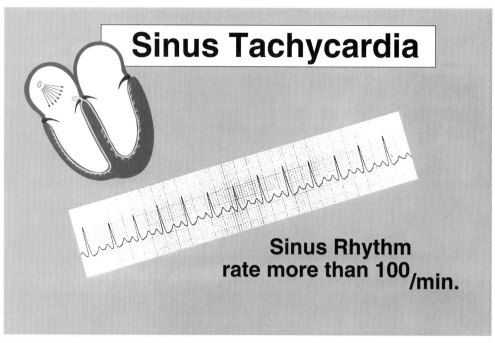

When the Sinus Node (SA Node) paces the heart at a rate greater than 100 per minute, this is *Sinus Tachycardia*.

NOTE: "Tachy" = fast; "cardia" = heart.

A rhythm originating in the Sinus Node (SA Node) is called Sinus Tachycardia when the rate is greater than _____ per minute.   100

Exercise will produce sympathetic stimulation of the SA Node; this is the most common cause of Sinus _____.   Tachycardia

NOTE: There are focal areas of automaticity in the heart known as **Automaticity Foci***. They are potential pacemakers that are capable of pacing in emergency situations. Under normal circumstances, these foci are electrically silent (that's why they are referred to as "potential" pacemakers).

* "*Automaticity foci*" refers to more than one "*automaticity focus*"; in fact, when the word "foci" is used alone, "*automaticity foci*" is understood. Foci is pronounced "FOE-sigh".

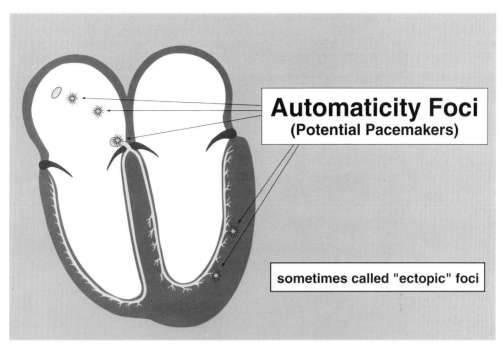

Automaticity Foci
(Potential Pacemakers)

sometimes called "ectopic" foci

Other potential pacemakers known as *automaticity foci* (also called "ectopic" foci) have the ability to pace (at their *inherent* rate) if normal SA Node pacemaking fails. They are in the atria, the ventricles, and the AV Junction.

If the SA Node ceases to function, one of the potential pacemakers, known as an automaticity focus, can assume pacemaking activity at its inherent _____ (one focus assumes pacing responsibility).

rate

The atria have automaticity _____ of potential pacemakers that are within the atrial conduction system (see page 97), and they are called *atrial automaticity foci.*

foci

NOTE: The proximal end of the AV Node has no automaticity foci, however the middle and distal regions of the AV Node, an area known as the *AV Junction* DOES HAVE automaticity foci that are called *Junctional automaticity foci.*

Purkinje fibers have automaticity foci, so there are foci of these potential _____ in the His Bundle, in the Bundle Branches and in all of their subdivisions, and they are called *ventricular automaticity foci.*

pacemakers

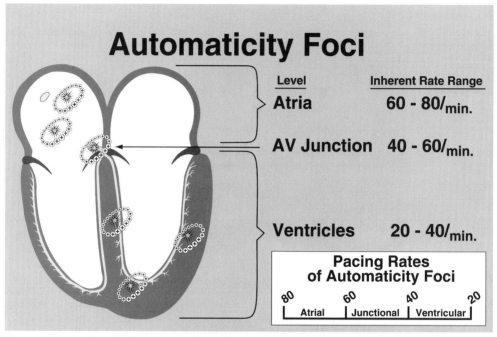

Automaticity Foci

Level	Inherent Rate Range
Atria	60 - 80/min.
AV Junction	40 - 60/min.
Ventricles	20 - 40/min.

Pacing Rates of Automaticity Foci

80	60	40	20
Atrial	Junctional	Ventricular

The automaticity foci of each "level" (the atria, the AV Junction, and the ventricles are each a "level") have a general range of pacemaking rate. Although all foci of a given level pace within a rate range, each individual automaticity focus has a precise *inherent rate* at which it paces.

Each automaticity focus of the atria has a specific inherent rate at which it paces, but its inherent rate falls within the range of ___ to 80 per minute.

60

The automaticity foci of the AV Junction all pace in the range of ___ to 60 per minute, but any single Junctional focus paces at its individual inherent rate.

40

Ventricular automaticity foci all pace in the ___ to 40 per minute range, but any specific ventricular focus has a distinct inherent rate of pacing.

20

SA Node overdrive-suppresses all lower foci (since all foci have slower inherent pacing rate)

SA Node

Overdrive Suppression

Atrial foci (inherent rate 60 – 80 per min.)

Junctional foci (inherent rate 40 – 60 per min.)

Ventricular foci (inherent rate 20 – 40 per min.)

Rapid pacemaking activity suppresses slower pacemaking activity – this is **overdrive suppression**, a fundamental characteristic of all automaticity centers.

NOTE: Overdrive suppression is characteristic of all centers of automaticity (including the SA Node and all automaticity foci). Simply stated: any automaticity center will overdrive-suppress* all others that have a slower inherent pacemaking rate.

The SA Node overdrive-suppresses the (slower) inherent pacemaking activity of all the automaticity _____ below it, providing the SA Node with the luxury   foci of not having to compete with slower pacemaking activity of lower automaticity foci.

In fact, once an automaticity focus actively begins pacing, it will overdrive-_____ all lower (slower) foci, including slower foci at the same level... ...eliminating any competition. Well Designed!

*When used as a verb, "overdrive-suppress" is hyphenated...so says my publisher.

67

OVERDRIVE SUPPRESSION
provides emergency backup pacing
at 3 separate levels

| Emergency Failsafe Pacing Mechanism |

SA Node
⇩
If Failure. . .
↳ **Atrial focus** assumes pacing responsibility.
⇩
If Failure. . .
↳ **AV Junctional focus** assumes pacing responsibility.
⇩
If Failure. . .
↳ **Ventricular focus** assumes pacing responsibility.

Overdrive suppression is the heart's failsafe pacing mechanism, providing three separate levels of backup pacing, utilizing automaticity foci in the atria, the ventricles, and the AV Junction.

NOTE: An automaticity focus actively pacing at its inherent rate, overdrive-suppresses all slower foci including slower foci at its own level.

Should normal pacing fail (pacemaker failure), a backup pacemaker (i.e. an automaticity focus from a lower level) – no longer overdrive-suppressed – will emerge to pace at its inherent rate, and it conveniently overdrive-suppresses potential pacemaking activity at all levels _____ it.   below

Therefore, an automaticity focus only emerges to function as a pacemaker when it is no longer _____-suppressed.   overdrive
For instance, in SA Node failure...

...a focus from a lower level – no longer overdrive-suppressed by regular pacing stimuli from above – can emerge to pace.
   Very well Designed!

Let's do that once again, slowly.

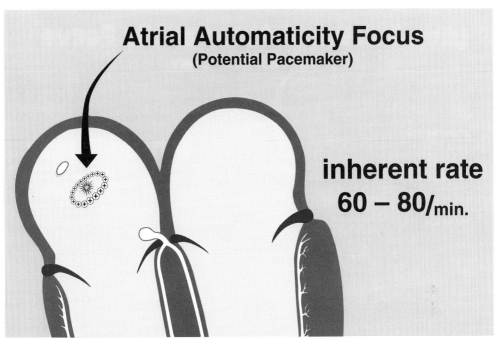

Atrial Automaticity Focus
(Potential Pacemaker)

**inherent rate
60 – 80/min.**

The atria have automaticity foci of potential pacemakers, any one of which can assume active pacemaking responsibility at its inherent rate range of about 60 to 80 per minute if normal pacemaking fails.

If the SA Node fails, an atrial automaticity _____ (within the atrial conduction system) may then assume active pacing responsibility and become the *dominant pacemaker*. (The last sentence on this page explains "dominant" pacemaker.)

focus

If SA Node pacing fails, an atrial automaticity focus can assume the active pacemaking responsibility at its inherent rate range of about 60 to ___ per minute (close to the SA Node's normal rate).

80

So without SA Node pacing, an atrial automaticity focus can emerge as an active backup pacemaker, and it becomes the *dominant pacemaker* by overdrive-suppressing all lower levels of foci, since they have slower_____ rates.

inherent

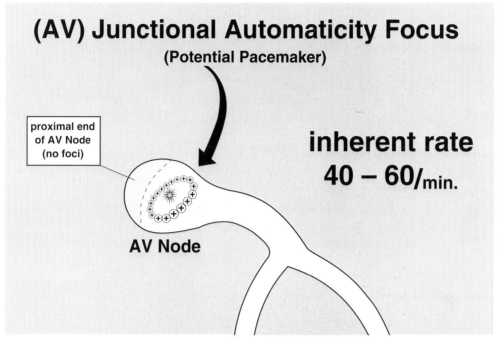

(AV) Junctional Automaticity Focus
(Potential Pacemaker)

proximal end
of AV Node
(no foci)

**inherent rate
40 – 60/min.**

AV Node

The AV Junction has automaticity foci (potential pacemakers), one of which will emerge to actively pace at its inherent rate range of 40 to 60 per minute if there is an <u>absence</u> of regular pacing stimuli progressing down from the atria.

NOTE: The AV Junction is that portion of the AV Node that has foci of automaticity. The proximal end of the AV node has no foci. The AV Junction has foci of automaticity that are referred to as "Junctional foci."

An automaticity focus in the AV Junction begins active backup pacing only in the absence of pacing stimuli coming down from the atria. Then, no longer overdrive-suppressed, it emerges to actively pace at its inherent _____ range of 40 to 60 per minute, and it overdrive-suppresses all   rate lower (slower) automaticity foci, becoming the dominant pacemaker.

An automaticity focus in the AV Junction, pacing at its inherent rate (____ to 60 per minute), produces an *idio-junctional** rhythm.   40

NOTE: An automaticity focus in the AV Junction (that is, a Junctional focus) emerges as the active pacemaker if it is no longer overdrive-suppressed by regular pacing stimuli from above. This can occur if the SA Node and all atrial foci fail. But wait, something else can prevent a Junctional focus from being depolarized by regular pacing stimuli from above. Next page!

* The prefix "idio" is of Greek origin, and it means "one's own." Idiojunctional is usually <u>not</u> hyphenated.

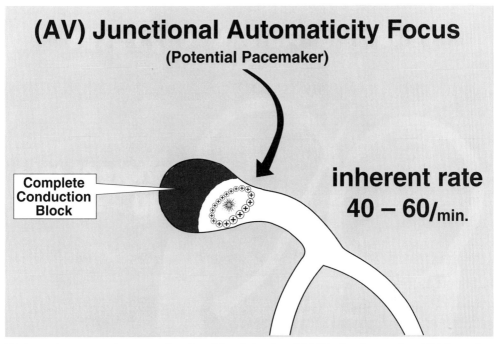

(AV) Junctional Automaticity Focus
(Potential Pacemaker)

Complete Conduction Block

inherent rate 40 – 60/min.

If there is a complete conduction block in the AV Node <u>above the AV Junction</u>, then no regular paced depolarization stimuli from above reach the automaticity foci in the AV Junction.

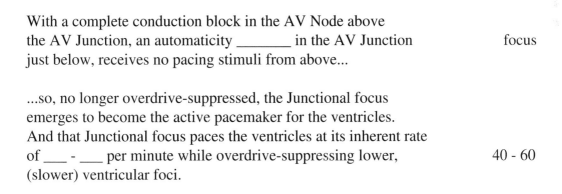

With a complete conduction block in the AV Node above the AV Junction, an automaticity _____ in the AV Junction just below, receives no pacing stimuli from above...

focus

...so, no longer overdrive-suppressed, the Junctional focus emerges to become the active pacemaker for the ventricles. And that Junctional focus paces the ventricles at its inherent rate of ___ - ___ per minute while overdrive-suppressing lower, (slower) ventricular foci.

40 - 60

NOTE: It is possible for the AV Junction (together with all its automaticity foci) to suffer a complete block. In that instance, only an automaticity focus in the Purkinje fibers of the ventricles can come to the rescue to pace the ventricles. Let's see how...

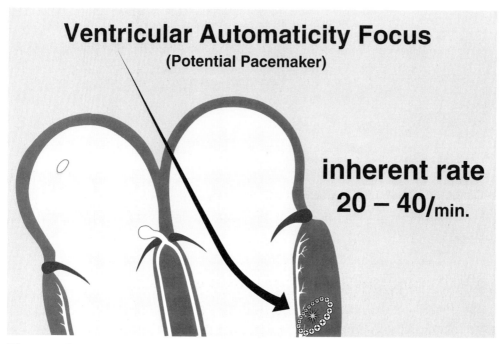

Ventricular Automaticity Focus
(Potential Pacemaker)

**inherent rate
20 – 40/min.**

The ventricles have automaticity foci (potential pacemakers), any one of which will assume pacing at its inherent rate range of 20 to 40 per minute if the usual overdrive suppression (due to regular pacing stimuli from above) is absent.

NOTE: Ventricular automaticity foci are composed of Purkinje cells within the Purkinje fibers. These pacemaking foci are in the His Bundle, the Bundle Branches, and all their subdivisions, since they are all are composed of Purkinje fibers.

Without overdrive suppression from above, a ventricular automaticity focus emerges to actively pace at its inherent rate range of ___ to 40 per minute; this is called an *idio-ventricular** rhythm.   20

NOTE: A ventricular focus emerges as the active ventricular pacemaker ONLY if it is no longer overdrive-suppressed by regular, paced stimuli from above. This occurs:
  • if all pacemaking centers above it have failed.
          -or-
  • if there is a complete block of conduction below the AV Node (including the AV Junction) that prevents any pacing stimulus above it (i.e., from the SA Node, an atrial focus, or a Junctional focus) from reaching the ventricles.

*Hyphenated here for ease of recognition, *idioventricular* should <u>not</u> be hyphenated.

OVERDRIVE SUPPRESSION
provides emergency backup pacing at 3 separate levels

Emergency Failsafe Pacing Mechanism

SA Node
⇩
If Failure...
↳ **Atrial focus** assumes pacing responsibility.
⇩
If Failure...
↳ **AV Junctional focus** assumes pacing responsibility.
⇩
If Failure...
↳ **Ventricular focus** assumes pacing responsibility.

Range of Inherent Pacing Rates of Automaticity Foci

80		60		40		20
	Atrial		Junctional		Ventricular	

If normal SA Node pacing fails, an automaticity focus in the atria, or the AV Junction, or even the ventricles (in that order) is available to assume the pacemaking responsibility at its own inherent rate. This provides three levels of backup pacing.

If the SA Node should cease pacing, an atrial automaticity focus can pace at its inherent rate range of 60 to 80 per minute; failing that, backup pacing by a focus in the AV Junction will assume the active _____ responsibility at its (slightly slower) inherent rate range of 40 - 60 per minute.   *pacing*

The ventricles can be paced by a ventricular automaticity focus at its _____ rate range of 20 to 40 per minute, if the focus   *inherent* is not regularly depolarized by paced stimuli. The lack of properly paced stimuli to the ventricular focus can be due to failure of all automaticity centers above, or due to an intervening complete conduction block that prevents pacing stimuli (from above) from conducting to the ventricles. (Such satisfaction understanding Nature!)

NOTE: In a physiological or pathological emergency, an automaticity focus may suddenly discharge at a rapid rate. This emergency rate (150 to 250 per minute) is approximately the same for foci of all levels.

Now let's try something real easy...

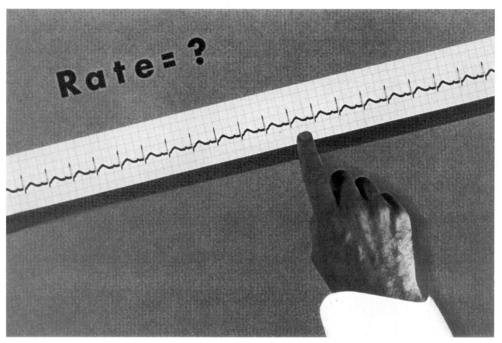

Our main objective is to rapidly determine the heart rate.

After finishing this chapter you will be able to determine
the _____ rapidly.   rate

No special devices, calculators, rulers, or awkward
mathematical computations are needed in order to
_____ the rate.   determine

NOTE: In emergency situations, you probably will not be able
to find, much less use a calculator; and you may not have the
presence of mind (or the time) to do mathematical calculations.

Observation alone can give us the _____.   rate

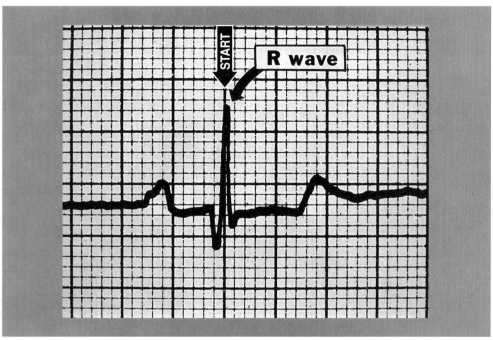

First: Find a specific R wave that peaks on a heavy black line (our "start" line).

To calculate rate, you should first look at the ___ waves.   R

Now find one that peaks on a heavy black line, and we will
call it the "_____" line.   start

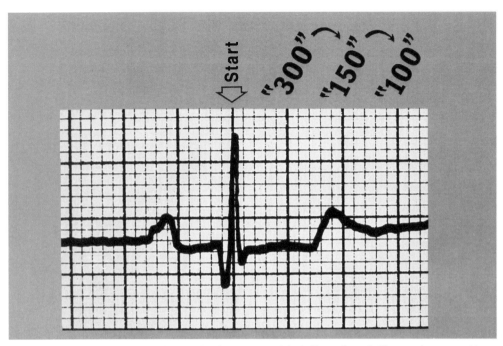

Next: Count off "300, 150, 100" for every thick line that follows the start line, naming each line as shown. Memorize these numbers.

An R wave peaks on a heavy black start line . . .
the <u>next</u> heavy black line is named "_____" . . . followed by   300
"_____" and "_____" for the next two heavy black lines.   150, 100

NOTE: The line that the R wave peaks upon is the start line; we only name the heavy lines that follow the start line.

The three lines following the start line (where the R wave falls) are named "_____, _____, _____" in succession.   300, 150, 100
(Say them out loud!)

Again!

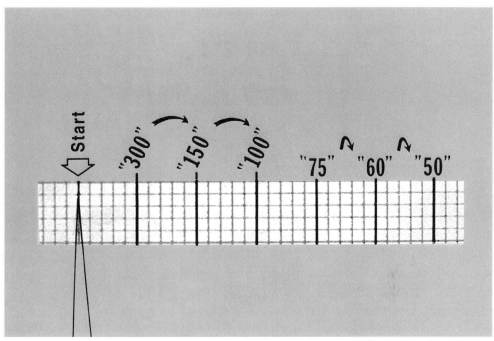

Then: Count off the next three lines after "300, 150, 100" as "75, 60, 50."

The next three lines after "300, 150, 100" are named
"_____, 60, 50."   75

Remember the next three lines together as:
"_____, _____, _____."   75, 60, 50

Once more out loud, please.

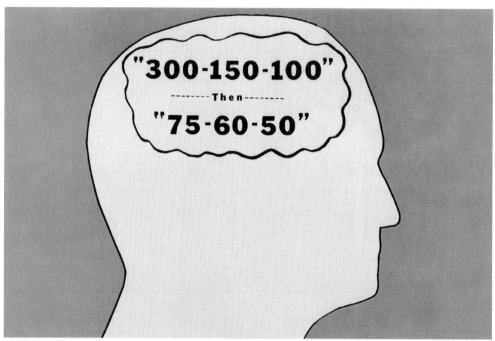

Now: Memorize these triplets until they are second nature. Make certain that you can *say* the triplets without using the picture.

These triplets, "300, 150, 100" and "75, 60, 50"
must be _____.   memorized

Be able to name the lines that follow the start line on which
an R wave _____; it is easy to remember them as   peaks
triplets, and so easy to use immediately. (Can hardly wait!)

Do not count those lines that follow the start line - NAME THEM
with the _____ as you go.   triplets

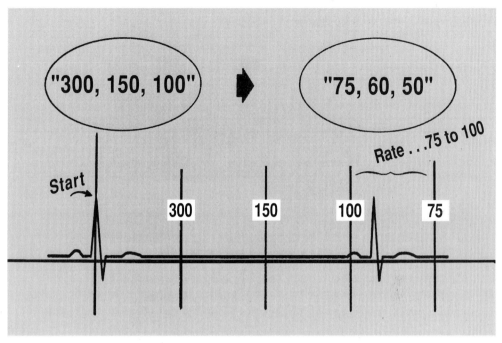

Where the next R wave falls, determines the rate. It's that simple.

Find an R wave peaked upon a heavy black (start) line,
then look for the _____ R wave.   next

Where the next R wave falls gives the _____.   rate
There is no need for mathematical computations.

If the next R wave falls on "75"...the rate is 75 per _____.   minute

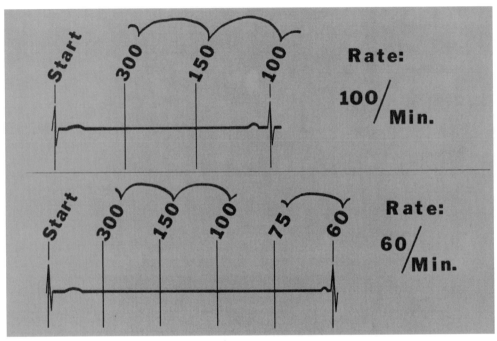

By knowing the triplets "300, 150, 100" then "75, 60, 50" you can merely look at an EKG and tell the approximate rate immediately.

The triplets are: first "_____, _____, _____."   300, 150, 100

          then "_____, _____, _____."   75, 60, 50

By simply naming the lines using the _____,   triplets
you can identify the rate immediately.

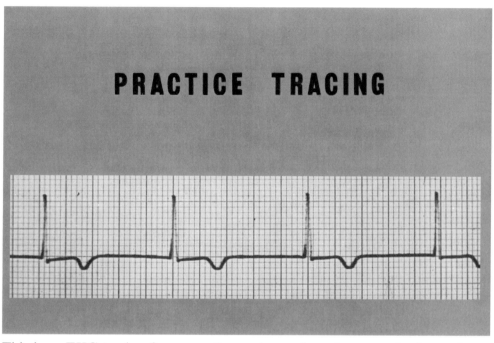

PRACTICE TRACING

This is an EKG tracing from a resting patient, whose heart rate is slower than the usual rate one would see with a Sinus Rhythm. Let's examine the rate.

The rate in the above tracing is about ____ per minute.   60

If you were told that this rhythm probably originated in an automaticity focus, by the rate alone, you would suspect the origin (pacemaker) to be in the ____ _____.   AV Junction

NOTE: This is indeed a rhythm originating in the AV Junction, and that's why you don't see P waves. This elderly woman has a very diseased heart. Her SA Node failed, then all the atrial automaticity foci failed. Fortunately, a Junctional focus came to the rescue. This natural pacing backup system is wonderfully effective.

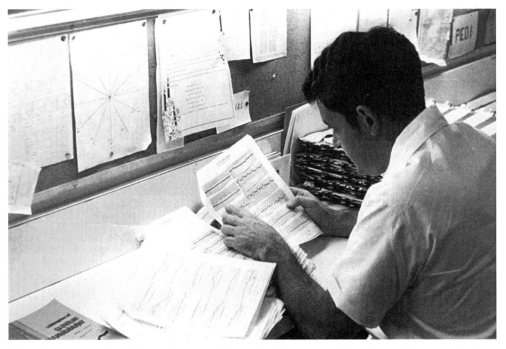

You do not need to depend on mathematical computations in order to calculate the rate. Observation alone will do it!

You can rapidly determine the rate on an EKG tracing
by _____ alone.   observation

There is no need to depend on annoying math or
calculators (where did I put that thing?) in order
to determine the _____.   rate

NOTE: You will always have your brain with you (at least until that time
when brain transplants would provide you with someone else's brain). Just
remember to name the lines that follow the *start* line using the triplets,
and say: "300, 150, 100" then "75, 60, 50."
Enough, enough . . . let's try it!

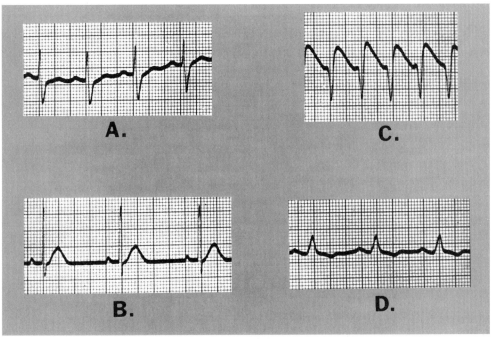

Now, let's determine the approximate rates of these EKG tracings.

A. _____   100

B. _____   60

C. _____   150 or so

D. _____   75

NOTE: As you may have discovered for yourself,
any prominent wave (like the S wave in example C.)
can be used to determine the rate.

The distance between the heavy black lines represents 1/300 min.

So two 1/300 min. units = 2/300 min. = 1/150 min.(or 150/min. rate)

and three 1/300 units = 3/300 = 1/100 min.(or 100/min. rate)

There is a logical explanation for the seemingly unusual rate determinations using the triplets.

NOTE: The unit of time (duration) between two heavy black lines is .2 sec., which is 1/300th of a minute.

The number of time units between five consecutive heavy black lines is ___.

4

So this represents 4/300 minute or a rate of _____ per minute.

75

Therefore if a heart contracts 75 times per minute, there will be a span equal to the distance between five heavy black lines between the _____ complexes.

QRS

NOTE: Reasonable instructors should not require students to master this page. As author, I have not personally memorized the text material on this page. Let's keep it simple and practical.

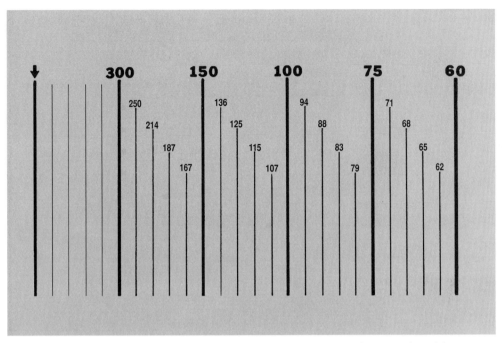

Although memorizing the fine line divisions is a tremendous undertaking, they provide for more precise rate determination. Most of us use a reference like that above, when determining very rapid rates.

NOTE: It is admittedly a great task to memorize the fine line subdivisions, but they are provided here and on page 311 as a convenient reference, should you need it.

NOTE: For rates less than sixty per minute, see the next few pages for a simple way to determine rate when you see a bradycardia.

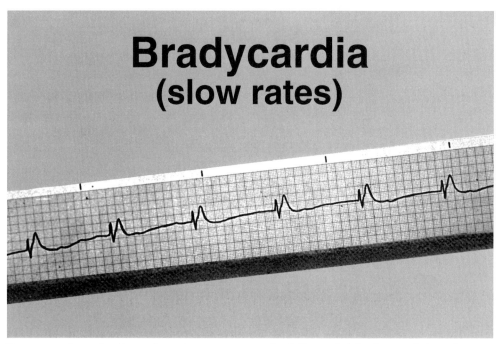

Bradycardia
(slow rates)

For very slow rhythms, here is an easy method for quickly determining the rate.

The proper term for slow heart rate is _____.   bradycardia

For very _____ rates you can use another method   slow
to determine the rate.

NOTE: The triplets give us a very large range of rates.
"300, 150, 100" then "75, 60, 50" means that you can
determine rates ranging from 300 to 50. Bradycardia
means a rate slower than 60 per minute. So...

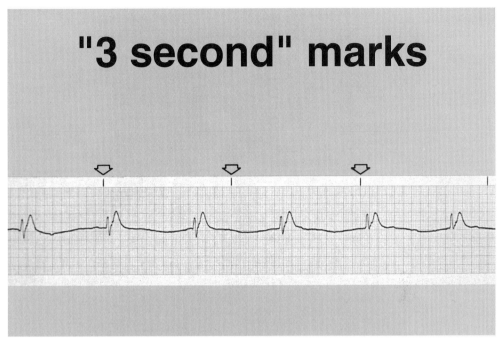

On the top margin of the EKG tracing there are small marks that signify the "three second" intervals.

There are small marks above the graph portion of the _____ tracing. Find a strip of EKG tracing and examine it.

EKG

Each of these marks signifies a three second _____.

interval

NOTE: Some EKG paper has 3 second intervals that are marked with a dot, circle, triangle, or a vertical line.

When an EKG machine is running, the span of paper between two of these "3 second interval" marks passes under the stylus needle in ___ _____.

3 seconds

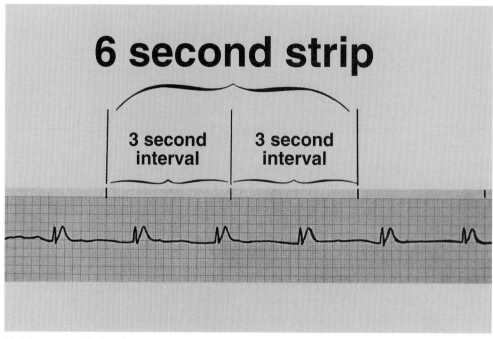

Taking two of the three second intervals, we have a 6 second strip.

NOTE: A three second interval is obviously the distance
between two consecutive 3 second interval marks.

Taking two of the three second intervals gives us a
6 second _____.   strip

This 6 second strip represents the amount of paper
used by the machine in six seconds (one-_____ of a minute).   tenth

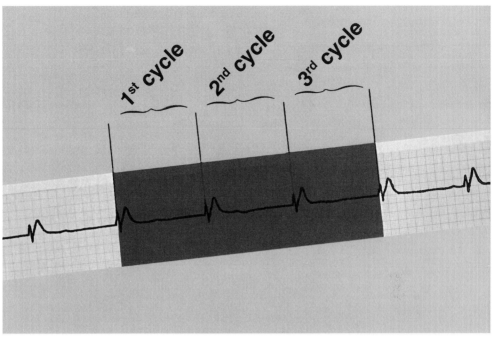

Count the number of complete (R wave to R wave) cycles in this 6 second strip. With marked bradycardia, there will be few cycles per 6 second strip.

The length of a cardiac _____ can be measured from a specific wave until the wave is repeated again.   cycle

So R wave to ___ wave gives us the duration (length) of one cardiac cycle.   R

Count the number of cycles in the 6 second _____.   strip

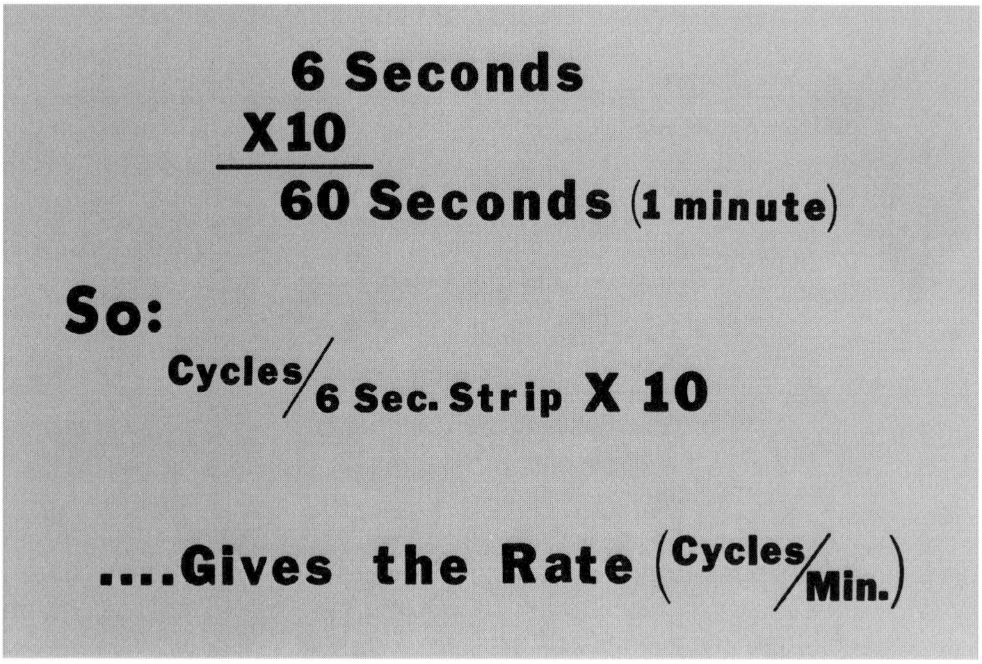

6 Seconds
X 10
_____
60 Seconds (1 minute)

So:

$$\text{Cycles}/\text{6 Sec. Strip} \; X \; 10$$

....Gives the Rate $\left(\text{Cycles}/\text{Min.}\right)$

The rate is obtained by multiplying the number of cycles in the 6 second strip by ten (10).

Ten of the 6 second strips equals one _____   minute
(time) recorded on EKG.

The number of cycles per minute is the _____.   rate

So cycles per 6 second strip multiplied by ___   10
equals the rate. Simple!

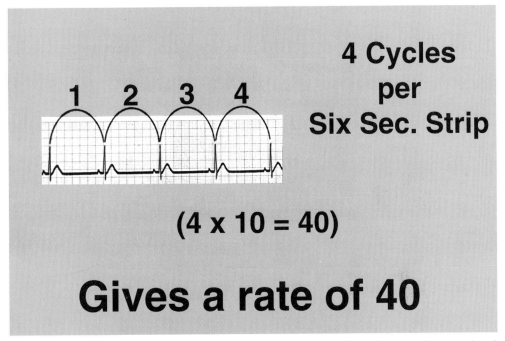

4 Cycles per Six Sec. Strip

1   2   3   4

(4 x 10 = 40)

Gives a rate of 40

You can just place a zero on the right of the number of cycles per 6 second strip, and you have the rate.

For very slow heart rates (bradycardia), you should first find a 6 second _____,   strip

. . . count the number of _____ in this strip,   cycles

. . . and multiply by ___ to get the rate.   10

NOTE: Multiplying by ten may be done by placing a zero on the right side of the number of cycles per 6 second strip. For instance, 5 cycles (per six second strip) gives a rate of 50.

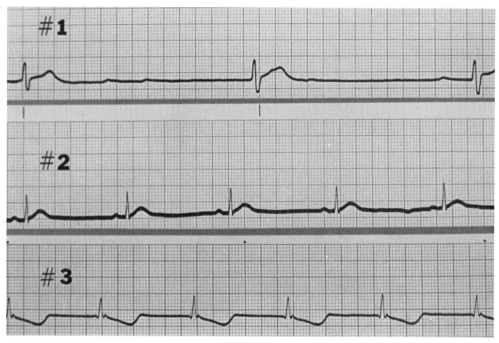

Let's determine the approximate rates of these EKG's.

Rates: No. 1. _____ per minute   20

        No. 2. _____ per minute   45

        No. 3. _____ per minute   50

NOTE: The general, average rates of irregular rhythms
may also be determined using this method.

Why don't you obtain some EKG tracings and amaze yourself and your friends
at how easily you can determine the rate.

NOTE: Review *Rate* by turning to the **Personal Quick Reference Sheets**
at the end of this book (pages 310 and 311).

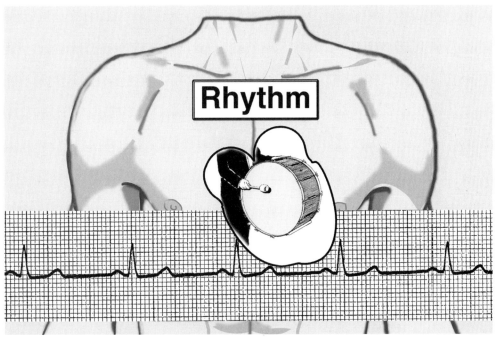

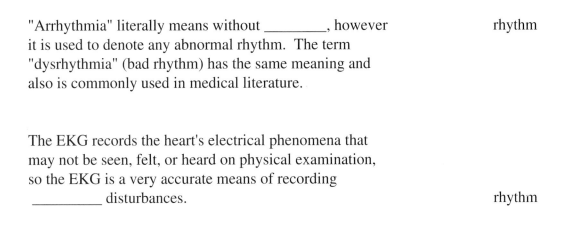

The EKG provides the most accurate means of identifying cardiac *arrhythmias* (abnormal rhythms), which can be diagnosed easily once we understand the electrophysiology of the heart.

"Arrhythmia" literally means without _____, however it is used to denote any abnormal rhythm. The term "dysrhythmia" (bad rhythm) has the same meaning and also is commonly used in medical literature.

rhythm

The EKG records the heart's electrical phenomena that may not be seen, felt, or heard on physical examination, so the EKG is a very accurate means of recording _____ disturbances.

rhythm

NOTE: To understand the arrhythmias you must first become familiar with the normal electrophysiology of the heart, including the normal conduction pathways.

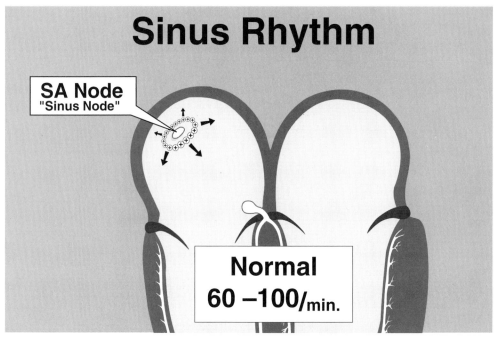

The SA Node generates a regular* Sinus Rhythm that paces the heart. Each pacemaker impulse from the SA Node (Sinus Node) spreads through both atria as an advancing wave of depolarization.

It is the automaticity of the Sinus Node (SA Node) which generates the regular* cadence of depolarization stimuli for pace-_____ activity.

making

Normally, the SA Node discharges regular pacing impulses (60 to 100 per minute) that depolarize the _____.

atria

NOTE: We know that the SA ("Sino-Atrial") Node is the same as the Sinus Node, so we understand that the stems "Sinus" and "Sino" imply SA Node origin.

*The term "regular" indicates a rhythm of constant rate. See next page...

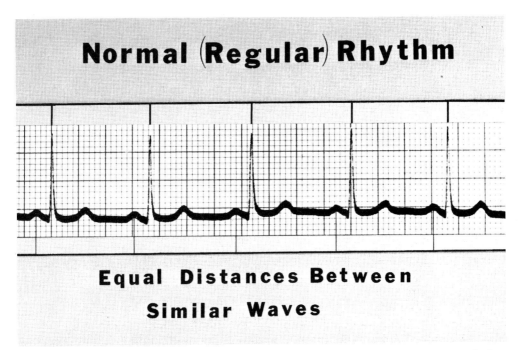

Normal (Regular) Rhythm

Equal Distances Between
Similar Waves

On EKG there is a consistent distance (duration) between similar waves during a normal, **regular** cardiac rhythm, because the automaticity of the SA Node precisely maintains a constant cycle duration between the pacing impulses that it generates.

NOTE: All automaticity foci pace with a regular rhythm.
This is a characteristic of all automaticity centers.

When the SA Node generates pacing impulses at a constant, unvarying rate, producing cycles of equal length, the rhythm of the heart is said to be _____. This characteristic   regular
pattern of regularity is typical of SA Node pacing*.

And because the sequence of depolarization is the same in each repeating cycle, there is a predictable pattern of regularity of all similar (name) waves. This makes any irregularities in _____ easy for you to spot on EKG.   rhythm

NOTE: We can visually scan an EKG and appreciate the repetitive continuity of a regular rhythm. But breaks in that continuity, like a pause, the presence of too-early (premature) beats, or sudden rate change, immediately catch our attention, warning us of a rhythm disturbance.

* In reality a Normal Sinus Rhythm varies imperceptibly with respiration.

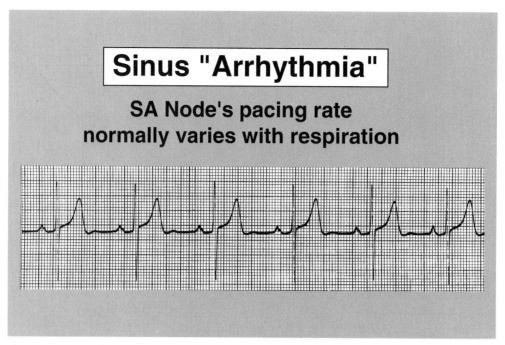

Sinus "Arrhythmia"

SA Node's pacing rate
normally varies with respiration

A normal physiological mechanism, *Sinus Arrhythmia,* sounds pathological ("arrhythmia" = abnormal rhythm), but it is functional in all humans at all times. The autonomic nervous system causes barely detectable rate changes in Sinus pacing that relate to the phases of respiration. This is not a true arrhythmia.

NOTE: Sinus Arrhythmia is a normal, but extremely minimal, increase in heart rate during inspiration, and an extremely minimal, decrease in heart rate during expiration.

Sinus Arrhythmia represents normal, minimal variations in the SA Node's pacing rate in association with the phases of _____.   respiration

NOTE: The slight increase in the heart rate is due to inspiration-activated *sympathetic* stimulation of the SA Node. The slight decrease in pacing rate is due to expiration-activated *parasympathetic* stimulation of the SA Node. You could have guessed that, because the SA Node's pacing rate is controlled by the two divisions of the Autonomic Nervous System.

NOTE: This variability of Sinus Rhythm is normal. In fact, if the heart rate variability is reduced, this is pathological and is a valuable indicator of increased mortality, particularly after infarction. Parameters of "Heart Rate Variability" are being established for determining patient prognosis for many types of heart disease.

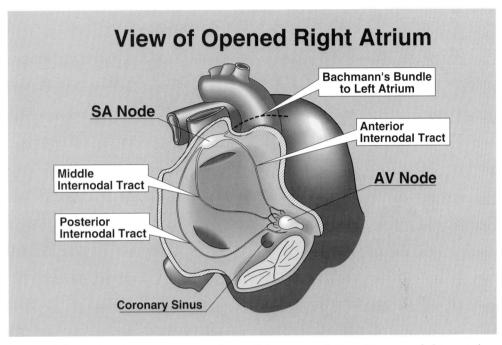

View of Opened Right Atrium

Bachmann's Bundle to Left Atrium

SA Node

Anterior Internodal Tract

Middle Internodal Tract

AV Node

Posterior Internodal Tract

Coronary Sinus

The atrial conduction system consists of three specialized *internodal tracts* in the right atrium (the *Anterior,* the *Middle,* and the *Posterior*), and one conduction tract known as *Bachmann's Bundle* that innervates the left atrium.

Three right atrial conduction pathways course from the SA Node to the AV Node (thus the term "Internodal"). They are the Anterior, the Middle, and the _____ Internodal Tracts.

Posterior

Bachmann's Bundle originates in the SA Node and distributes depolarization to the left _____.

atrium

Rapid depolarization passing through the atrial conduction system does not record on EKG; however, depolarization of the atrial myocardium produces a ___ wave on EKG.

P

NOTE: Just as ventricular automaticity foci are within the ventricular Purkinje fibers, similarly, atrial automaticity foci are within the specialized atrial conduction system. Because there is a concentration of merging atrial conduction tracts in the immediate region of the AV Node near the *coronary sinus**, considerable automaticity activity originates in that area.

*The heart's own venous drainage (i.e., from the myocardium) empties into the right atrium via the coronary sinus.

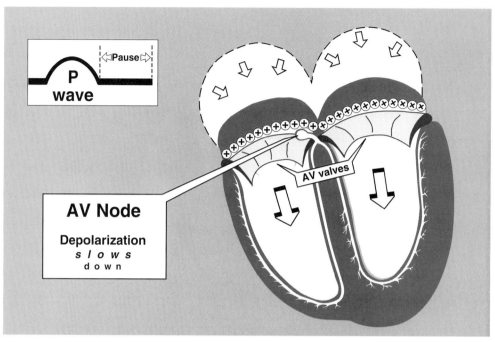

When the stimulus of depolarization (passing down from the atria) reaches the AV Node, the stimulus s l o w s in the AV Node producing a pause on EKG.

Atrial depolarization eventually reaches the AV Node, but conduction of depolarization slows within the AV Node, recording a _____ on EKG.   pause

This pause (during which blood from the atria passes into the ventricles) is represented by the horizontal piece of baseline between the P wave and the _____ complex.   QRS

NOTE: The AV Node is named for its position between the Atria and the Ventricles (thus "AV"). The proximal end of the AV Node has no automaticity foci. However, the remainder of the AV Node, an area known as the AV Junction, does have automaticity foci. These foci are essential for backup pacing should there be a total failure of all pacemaking activity from above (SA Node as well as atrial foci), or if a complete conduction block of the proximal end of the AV Node occurs, preventing all (SA Node or atrial foci) pacing stimuli from being conducted to the ventricles.

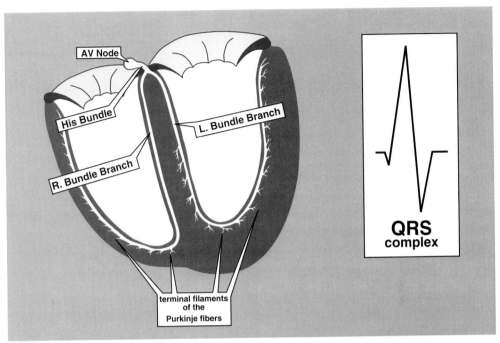

After passing (s l o w l y) through the AV Node, depolarization proceeds rapidly through the His Bundle, Bundle Branches and their subdivisions, and through the terminal Purkinje filaments to distribute depolarization to the ventricles. Ventricular depolarization produces a QRS complex on the EKG.

NOTE: The His Bundle and the Bundle Branches are "bundles" of rapidly conducting Purkinje fibers. Depolarization passing through the Purkinje fibers of the ventricular conduction system is too weak to record on EKG; this is a form of "concealed" conduction.

After c r e e p i n g through the AV Node, depolarization shifts gears and races through the His _____, and...   Bundle

...through the Right and Left Bundle Branches and their subdivisions to rapidly transmit depolarization via the terminal Purkinje filaments to the endocardial surface of the _____ myocardium.   ventricular

When the ventricular myocardium depolarizes, it produces a _____ complex on EKG.   QRS

NOTE: The Purkinje fibers of the ventricular conduction system contain automaticity foci (you knew that already).

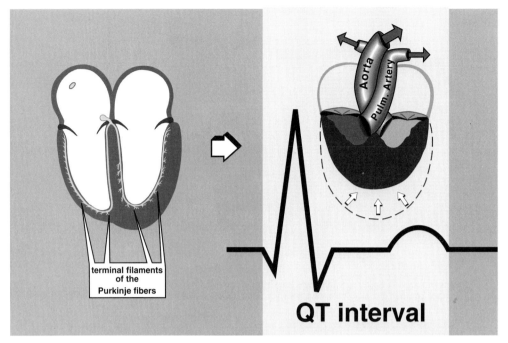

QT interval

The Purkinje fibers of the ventricular conduction system rapidly conduct depolarization away from the AV Node to the endocardial surface of the ventricles; when the ventricles depolarize, it produces a QRS complex on EKG.

NOTE: Ventricular depolarization begins midway down the interventricular septum where the Left Bundle Branch is first to produce fine terminal filaments. So left-to-right depolarization of the septum occurs immediately before the rest of the ventricular myocardium depolarizes.

Ventricular depolarization initiates ventricular contraction, which persists (through both phases of repolarization) to the end of the __ wave.   T

Ventricular contraction begins and ends during the ____ interval.   QT

NOTE: Repolarization of the Purkinje fibers takes longer than ventricular repolarization. That is, the end of the T wave marks the end of ventricular repolarization; however, repolarization of the Purkinje fibers terminates a little later — beyond the end of the T wave. The final phase of Purkinje repolarization may record a small hump, the *U wave* (following the T wave), on EKG.

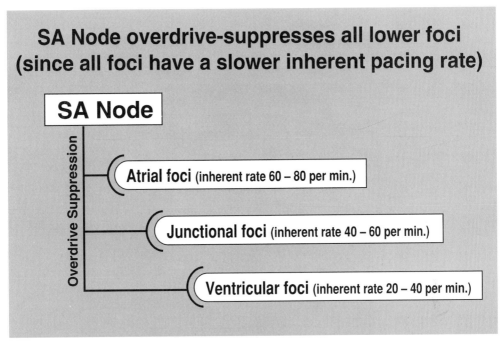

There are three levels of automaticity foci (atria, AV Junction, and ventricles) which can provide backup pacemaker responsibility if pacing activity fails. The foci of each level have a characteristic inherent rate range giving the SA Node a failsafe hierarchy of three levels of backup pacing.

Each level of automaticity foci has a consistent range of _____ rate. *inherent*

NOTE: The SA Node and all automaticity foci are centers of automaticity ("automaticity centers"), which means that they can generate regular pacing stimuli.

Overdrive suppression allows the automaticity center with the fastest rate to be the _____ pacemaker (no competition). *dominant*

Should the highest pacemaking center fail, an automaticity focus from the next highest level (no longer overdrive-suppressed) emerges to actively pace at its inherent rate, and it then becomes the dominant pacemaker by overdrive-suppressing all automaticity _____ below it. *foci*

NOTE: A very "irritable" automaticity focus may suddenly pace rapidly.

Arrhythmias

- **Irregular Rhythms (page 103)**
- **Escape   (page 108)**
- **Premature Beats   (page 118)**
- **Tachy–arrhythmias   (page 141)**
- **Heart Blocks   (page 165)**

The arrhythmias can be divided into a few general categories according to the mechanism of origin of the arrhythmia. The best students, I've noticed, apply index tabs to the pages that begin each arrhythmia category (see above); try it — you will find it very helpful!

NOTE: Although arrhythmia literally means "without rhythm," generally it is used to denote any rhythm disturbance, that is, any variance from a Normal Sinus Rhythm. Some authors prefer the term "dysrhythmia" rather than arrhythmia.

NOTE: The illustration is a simplified arrhythmia classification that is categorized according to the mechanism of origin, so the arrhythmias will be easy to understand.

The underlying mechanisms that are basic to the heart's function are very satisfying to learn. But more importantly, conceptual understanding of the basic mechanisms facilitates and perpetuates your knowledge. Don't memorize patterns; your knowledge will be vital to others! Lasting knowledge results from understanding.

Irregular Rhythms

- **Wandering Pacemaker**
- **Multifocal Atrial Tachycardia**
- **Atrial Fibrillation**

The very irregular rhythms presented in this section are usually caused by multiple, active automaticity sites.

Rhythms that lack a constant duration between paced cycles are said to be _____.

irregular

NOTE: The term "irregularly irregular" is an old designation that describes an irregular and chaotic rhythm that has no predictable recurring pattern.

NOTE: In some hearts with structural pathology or hypoxia, automaticity foci may have a malfunction known as **entrance block** whereby any incoming depolarization is blocked, "protecting" them from passive depolarization by any other source. The "protection" is not healthy, because by being insensitive to passive depolarization they cannot be overdrive-suppressed, *while their own automaticity is still conducted to surrounding tissue.*

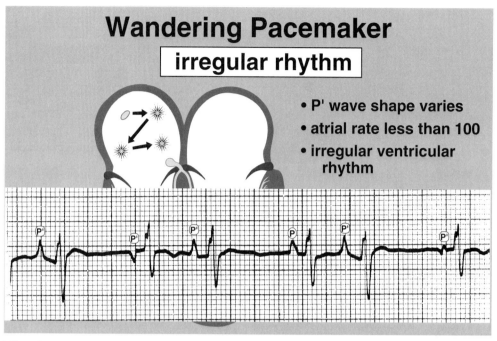

Wandering Pacemaker

irregular rhythm

- P' wave shape varies
- atrial rate less than 100
- irregular ventricular rhythm

Wandering Pacemaker is an irregular rhythm produced by the pacemaker activity wandering from the SA Node to nearby atrial automaticity foci. This produces cycle length variation as well as variation in the shape of the P' waves. The overall rate, however, is within the normal range.

NOTE: The P' (pronounced "P prime") wave represents atrial depolarization by an automaticity focus.

NOTE: Each automaticity focus has a specific inherent rate at which it paces. In a given lead, each atrial automaticity focus produces its own morphological signature, that is, it produces a P' wave of a specific shape related to the anatomical location of that focus within the atria.

Wandering Pacemaker is an irregular rhythm (normal rate range); the pacemaking activity wanders from the SA Node to _____ foci...   atrial

...so the cycle lengths vary, and __ wave morphology (shape) varies   P' as the pacemaking center moves.

NOTE: Should the rate increase into the tachycardia range (greater than 100 per minute), this becomes *Multifocal Atrial Tachycardia*. Next page please...

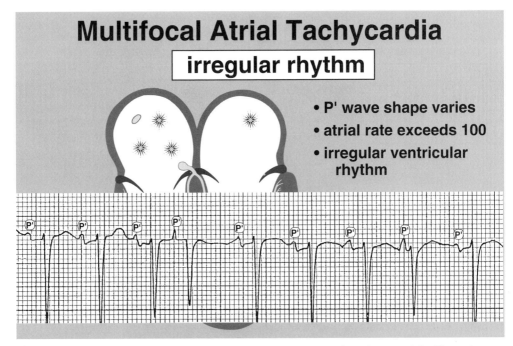

Multifocal Atrial Tachycardia
irregular rhythm

- **P' wave shape varies**
- **atrial rate exceeds 100**
- **irregular ventricular rhythm**

Multifocal Atrial Tachycardia (MAT) is a rhythm of patients with Chronic Obstructive Pulmonary Disease (COPD). The heart rate is over 100 per minute with P' waves of various shapes, since three or more atrial foci are involved.

In MAT, we can recognize a P' wave from a particular _____ focus by its morphological signature, i.e., P' waves from the same focus look the same in a given lead.

atrial

NOTE: MAT is an arrhythmia of patients who are very ill* with COPD. The atrial automaticity foci are also ill, showing early signs of "protective" entrance block by a developing a resistance to being overdrive-suppressed. That is why no single fucus achieves pacemaking dominance.

Because of the multifocal origin of MAT, each individual atrial focus paces at its own inherent _____, but the total, combined "normal" pacing of multiple unsuppressed foci produces a rapid, irregular rhythm...

rate

...and in a given lead, each focus produces P' waves with a specific morphological signature, i.e., __ waves of a distinct shape (note the variety of P' waves in the illustration). And remember, this is a tachycardia.

P'

* MAT is sometimes associated with digitalis toxicity in patients with heart disease.

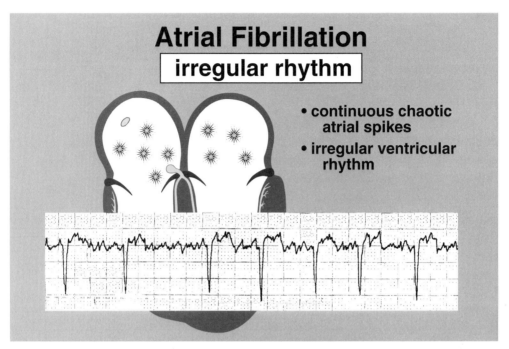

Atrial Fibrillation
irregular rhythm

- **continuous chaotic atrial spikes**
- **irregular ventricular rhythm**

Atrial Fibrillation is caused by the continuous, rapid-firing of multiple atrial automaticity foci. No single impulse depolarizes the atria completely, and only an occasional atrial depolarization gets through the AV Node to stimulate the ventricles, producing an irregular ventricular (QRS) rhythm.

NOTE: Atrial Fibrillation is NOT an arrhythmia of healthy, young individuals. It is the result of multiple "irritable" atrial foci with *entrance block,* pacing rapidly. These multiple atrial foci are insensitive to overdrive suppression, so they all pace at once. What chaos!

During Atrial Fibrillation no single impulse completely depolarizes both _____, so there are no true P waves, only a rapid series of tiny, erratic spikes on EKG.

atria

Only the occasional atrial impulse gets through the AV Node to initiate a ____ complex. The *irregular ventricular response* may result in either a slow or rapid ventricular rate, but it is always irregular.

QRS

NOTE: You must ALWAYS determine and document the general ventricular rate in Atrial Fibrillation (QRS's per six second strip times 10).

PRACTICE TRACING

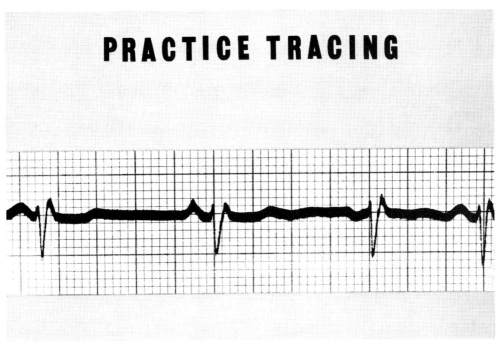

This tracing was monitored from a patient with an irregular pulse.

This practice tracing has an irregular rhythm in which
we see discernible ___ waves, so we know that it is not
Atrial Fibrillation.

P'

The "P" waves are not identical, and the rate does not gradually
increase and gradually decrease, so we immediately know that
this is not _____ Arrhythmia.

Sinus

The rate is less than 100 (which rules out MAT), the rhythm
is irregular, and the P' waves are of different shapes. This is
most likely _____ Pacemaker.

Wandering

Easy, isn't it!

NOTE: Just to solidify your knowledge of these irregular rhythms,
maybe you should review the illustrations on the last few pages.

Escape

Escape Rhythm - an automaticity focus escapes overdrive suppression to <u>pace</u> at its inherent rate:
- Atrial Escape Rhythm
- Junctional Escape Rhythm
- Ventricular Escape Rhythm

Escape Beat - an automaticity focus <u>transiently</u> escapes overdrive suppression to emit <u>one</u> <u>beat</u>:
- Atrial Escape Beat
- Junctional Escape Beat
- Ventricular Escape Beat

"**Escape**" describes the response of an automaticity focus to a pause in the pacemaking activity.

The SA Node's regular pacing overdrive-suppresses all automaticity foci, but a brief pause in SA Node pacing permits an automaticity _____ to escape overdrive suppression.

focus

If SA Node pacing ceases entirely, an automaticity focus will escape to pace at its inherent _____, thereby producing an *Escape Rhythm*. We will, however, need to identify the focus (atrial, Junctional, or ventricular) that escapes to actively pace.

rate

If the pause in pacing is brief (one cycle missed), an automaticity focus may _____ to emit a single *Escape Beat*. So, we will need to identify that focus (atrial, Junctional, or ventricular).

escape

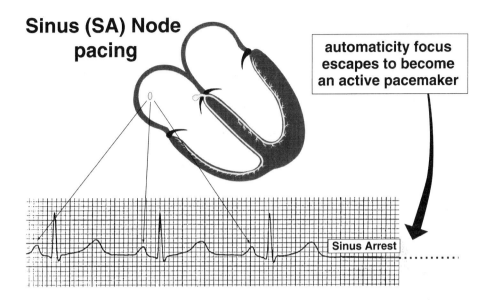

Sinus (SA) Node pacing

automaticity focus escapes to become an active pacemaker

Sinus Arrest

Sinus Arrest occurs when a very sick SA Node ceases pacemaking completely. But the heart's efficient failsafe mechanism provides three separate levels of automaticity foci for backup pacemaking. Divine Design.

NOTE: With a Sinus Arrest, the SA Node ceases pacing; then, absent overdrive suppression by the SA Node, an automaticity focus (with the fastest inherent pacing rate) escapes to become an active pacemaker; and by overdrive-suppressing all foci below, it becomes the dominant pacemaker.

NOTE: *An automaticity focus is overdrive-suppressed if regularly depolarized by a pacing rate faster than its own inherent pacing rate.* But if an automaticity focus is not overdrive-suppressed – regardless of the cause – it escapes to initiate its own pacemaking activity.

NOTE: *Each specific focus has its own individual, inherent rate of pacing.* However, the inherent pacing rates of all automaticity foci of a given level (for example, the inherent rates of all Junctional foci) are within a rate range.

NOTE: With a Sinus Arrest, the SA Node ceases pacing, so absent overdrive suppression from above, an automaticity focus escapes to produce an Escape Rhythm. However with Sinus Block, the SA Node misses one pacing cycle, producing a transient pause. So an automaticity focus escapes to emit an Escape Beat, which really represents the first beat of the attempt by the focus to pace, but the return of SA Node pacing overdrive-suppresses it again.

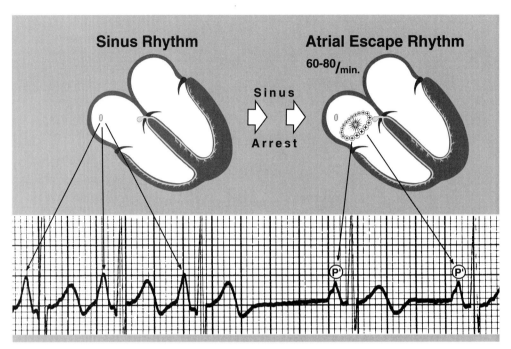

With Sinus Arrest an atrial focus quickly escapes overdrive suppression
to become the dominant pacemaker at its inherent rate. This is an
Atrial Escape Rhythm.

With a Sinus Arrest, an automaticity focus in the highest
level of foci, the _____, escapes overdrive suppression   atria
to become an active pacemaker at its inherent rate range
of 60 to 80 per minute.

An Atrial Escape Rhythm originates in an atrial automaticity
focus, so the P' waves are not identical to the previous P waves
that were produced by the _____. (See illustration.)   SA Node

NOTE: The active atrial automaticity focus overdrive-suppresses all lower,
slower foci to become the dominant pacemaker. It also paces at its inherent
rate, which differs from (i.e., slower than) the previous Sinus rate. See
illustration.

Atrial _____ Rhythm describes the natural mechanism that   Escape
initiates the rhythm, and I doubt that it needs repeating.

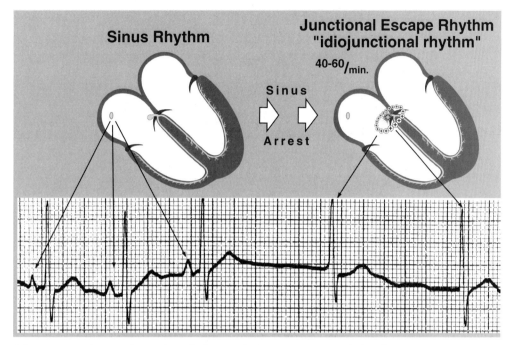

Sinus Rhythm

Junctional Escape Rhythm "idiojunctional rhythm"

40-60/min.

Sinus

Arrest

Absent regular pacing stimuli from above, an automaticity focus in the AV Junction may escape overdrive suppression to become an active pacemaker producing a *Junctional Escape Rhythm* at its inherent rate range: 40 to 60 per minute.

NOTE: A Junctional focus escapes the influence of overdrive suppression if there is a Sinus Arrest and the atrial foci also fail to function properly...

...or if there is a complete conduction block in the proximal end of the AV Node. In either case, the Junctional focus is not regularly stimulated by pacing depolarizations from above.

When a Junctional focus is not overdrive-suppressed, it actively paces, producing a Junctional Escape Rhythm, and it becomes the dominant pacemaker of the ventricles at a rate ranging from 40 to ___ per minute (it's also called an "idiojunctional rhythm")*.　　　60
.

A Junctional Escape Rhythm usually conducts mainly to the ventricles, producing a series of lone ____ complexes. But　　　QRS see the next page for an interesting exception.

* Sometimes the inherent Junctional pacing rate may accelerate beyond its usual range to produce an *Accelerated Idiojunctional Rhythm*.

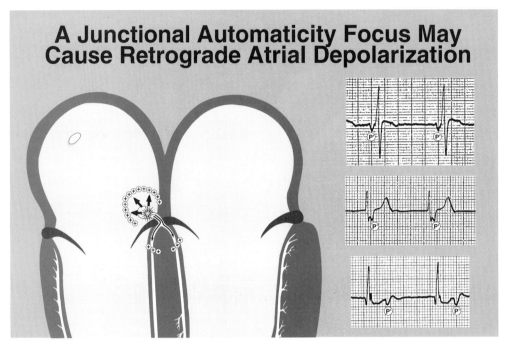

A Junctional Automaticity Focus May Cause Retrograde Atrial Depolarization

Because each Junctional automaticity focus is located within the AV Node, each depolarization stimulus originating there will conduct to the ventricles as expected, but the paced stimuli may also (unexpectedly) depolarize the atria from below (retrograde) producing *inverted* P' waves on EKG.

When a Junctional focus paces an escape rhythm, every paced stimulus will depolarize the ventricles in a normal fashion, but the pacing may also depolarize the atria from below in a *retrograde* fashion, producing _____ P' waves on EKG.   inverted

NOTE: The AV Node conducts very slowly, so depolarization from a Junctional focus may delay <u>either</u> ventricular depolarization or retrograde atrial depolarization (if present)...

...as a result, if there is retrograde atrial depolarization from a Junctional focus, it may record on EKG with one of these three patterns:

- retrograde (inverted) P' wave immediately before each QRS
- retrograde (inverted) P' wave after each QRS
- retrograde (inverted) P' wave buried within each QRS (not shown in illustration)

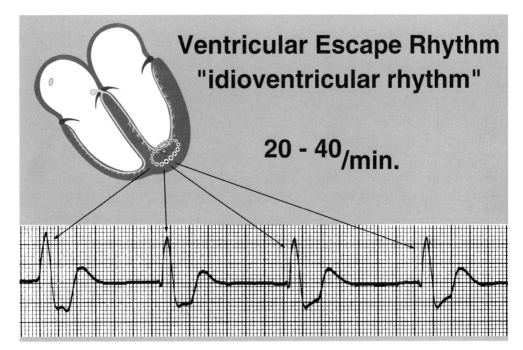

Ventricular Escape Rhythm "idioventricular rhythm"

20 - 40/min.

A *Ventricular Escape Rhythm* occurs when a ventricular automaticity focus is not regularly stimulated by paced depolarizations from above, so it escapes overdrive suppression to emerge as the ventricular pacemaker with an inherent rate in the range of 20 to 40 per minute* (so it is also called an "idioventricular rhythm"). Notice the enormous ventricular complexes.

NOTE: Ventricular Escape Rhythm usually results from one of two mechanisms:

•Total failure of the SA Node and all automaticity foci above the ventricles is a rare and grave condition, (previously called "downward displacement of the pacemaker"). In extremis, a ventricular focus escapes to become the active ventricular pacemaker in a final, futile attempt to sustain life.

•If there is a complete conduction block high in the ventricular conduction system (but below the AV Node), the ventricular foci will not be stimulated by the regular pacing stimuli from above, so a ventricular focus escapes to pace the ventricles at its inherent rate.

NOTE: Pacing from a ventricular focus is often so slow that blood flow to the brain is significantly reduced to the point of unconsciousness (syncope). This is *Stokes-Adams Syndrome*. This unconscious patient needs to have his (or her) airway monitored and maintained...constantly.

* Should this accelerate above the inherent rate range, it becomes an *Accelerated Idioventricular Rhythm.*

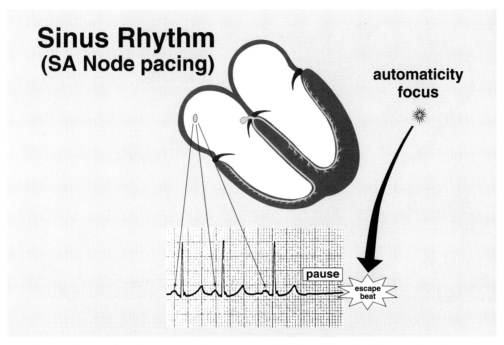

Sinus Rhythm
(SA Node pacing)

automaticity
focus

pause

escape
beat

During a Sinus Rhythm, a transient *Sinus Block* makes the SA Node miss
a pacing stimulus (one missed cycle), so an atrial automaticity focus escapes its
overdrive suppression to emit an *Escape Beat*.

With a transient Sinus Block, an unhealthy SA Node misses
one pacing stimulus. This missed cycle produces a _____   pause
during which the heart is electrically silent.

If this pause is long enough (see NOTE below), then an
automaticity focus will "escape" _____ suppression.   overdrive

NOTE: If there is a "sufficient" pause — longer than the
inherent (pacing) cycle length of an automaticity focus — that focus
will "escape" the SA Node's overdrive suppression to emit a stimulus*.

If the SA Node misses only one cycle, it will then resume pacing
and the SA Node's overdrive suppression of all automaticity
_____ resumes as well.   foci

* If you don't understand the NOTE, don't worry. Just be aware of the escape mechanism.

114

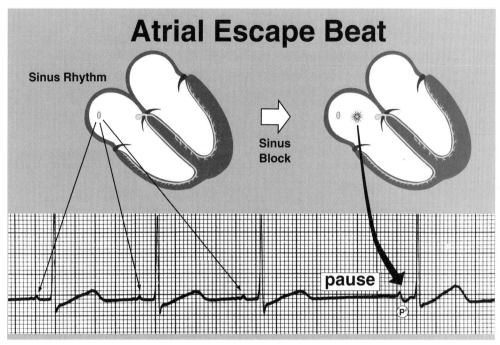

Atrial Escape Beat

Sinus Rhythm

Sinus Block

pause

P'

A transient Sinus Block of one pacemaking stimulus (SA Node misses one cycle) is a sufficient pause for an atrial automaticity focus to escape overdrive suppression and emit an *Atrial Escape Beat*. Notice that the P' wave differs from the Sinus-generated P waves.

A transient Sinus Block can prevent the ___ _____ from discharging one pacemaking stimulus, thus producing a pause of electrical silence for one pacing cycle.

SA Node

This pause, resulting from one missed SA Node pacing cycle, is sufficient enough to suspend the overdrive suppression of an atrial automaticity _____ and...

focus

...the atrial focus then escapes to emit a single stimulus; this is an Atrial Escape Beat (on EKG a different looking P'). But, when the SA Node resumes pacing, the atrial focus will be _____-suppressed again.

overdrive

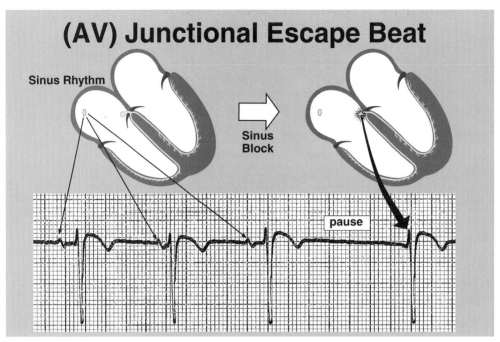

(AV) Junctional Escape Beat

Sinus Rhythm

Sinus Block

pause

An unhealthy SA Node that suffers a transient Sinus Block misses one pacing cycle. This pause can induce a Junctional automaticity focus to escape overdrive suppression and emit a *Junctional Escape Beat*.

If the SA Node suffers a transient Sinus Block, it misses one pacing cycle, so a sufficient _____ results and...   pause

...absent any atrial focal response, a Junctional automaticity focus will escape overdrive _____ to emit a   suppression
Junctional Escape Beat.

The depolarization stimulus emitted by the Junctional focus passes down the ventricular conduction _____ to depolarize the   system
ventricles in a normal fashion, so a normal QRS complex results. Then the SA Node resumes pacemaking, overdrive-suppressing the Junctional focus.

NOTE: A single Junctional Escape Beat may produce retrograde atrial depolarization that records an inverted P' immediately before the QRS or an inverted P' after the QRS.

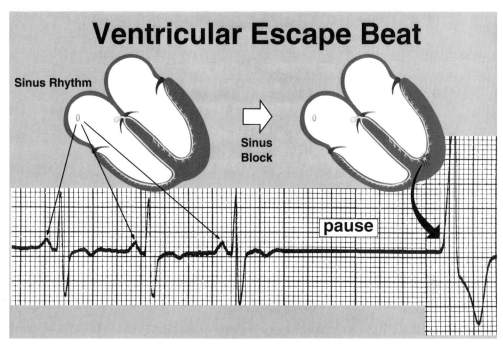

Ventricular Escape Beat

Sinus Rhythm

Sinus Block

pause

A *Ventricular Escape Beat* originates in a ventricular automaticity focus when it is no longer overdrive-suppressed by regular pacing stimuli from above. A ventricular focus typically produces this enormous ventricular (QRS) complex.

A ventricular automaticity _____ can escape overdrive suppression when it is not stimulated by pacemaking activity from above for at least one - maybe two cycles.   focus

It seems a little unusual that the SA Node as well as all of the atrial foci and all the Junctional _____ would fail simultaneously. How then is it, that Ventricular Escape Beats are not so rare? Here's how...   foci

NOTE: Cardiac parasympathetic innervation inhibits the SA Node AND ALSO inhibits the atrial and Junctional foci too (see illustration, page 57), but not the ventricular foci. Therefore, a burst of excessive parasympathetic activity depresses the SA Node (producing a pause) and also depresses the atrial and Junctional foci, which leaves only the ventricular foci to respond to the pause. So a ventricular automaticity focus escapes overdrive suppression and discharges, depolarizing the ventricles, producing an enormous ventricular complex. Such a burst of excessive parasympathetic activity is usually transient, so the SA Node resumes its pacemaking activity.

Premature Beats

Premature Beat - an irritable focus spontaneously fires a single stimulus:

- **Atrial Premature Beat**

- **Junctional Premature Beat**

- **Ventricular Premature Beat**

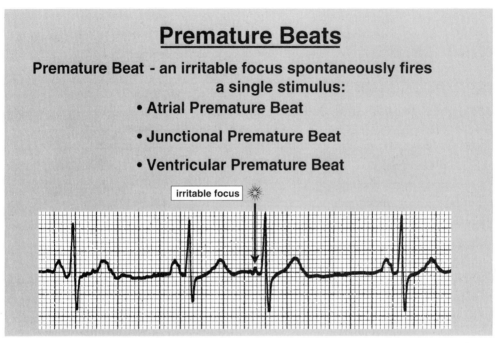

irritable focus

A *premature beat* (premature stimulus) originates in an <u>irritable</u> automaticity focus that fires spontaneously, producing a beat (on EKG we see evidence of a depolarization) earlier than expected in the rhythm.

NOTE: Those things that make *you* irritable can do the same to an atrial or Junctional automaticity focus. Quickly peek at the next page and you'll see.

A premature beat, like a premature baby, appears earlier than _____.
expected

When we see a premature beat, we recognize that it was fired by an irritable automaticity _____, so we need to identify the focus (atrial, Junctional, or ventricular).
focus

NOTE: Ventricular automaticity foci are the world's most sensitive O_2 sensors. When they sense low O_2, they become irritable...and they react!

NOTE: Premature beats can cause peculiarities in the rhythm that may mimic more serious problems such as pathological conduction blocks. While some premature beats are not serious, others are a dire warning – we'll explore them all. You should be cautious and know the difference – lives will depend on it! Understanding the basics provides answers and also facilitates practical comprehension for immediate recognition.

Atrial and **Junctional** foci become irritable because of:

- adrenaline (epinephrine) released by adrenal glands

- increased sympathetic stimulation*

- presence of caffeine, amphetamines, cocaine,
  or other β_1 receptor stimulants

- excess digitalis, some toxins, occasionally ethanol
- hyperthyroidism
  (direct stimulation plus heart oversensitive
  to adrenergic stimulants)

. . . and to some extent, low O_2
  and stretch

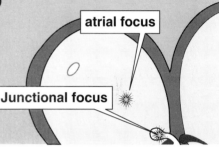

atrial focus

Junctional focus

* decreasing or blocking parasympathetic effects
may accomplish this.

An *automaticity focus in the atria or in the AV Junction* may become **irritable** and spontaneously fire an impulse or even suddenly pace very fast. The cause of irritability in atrial and Junctional foci is usually adrenergic substances (p. 56).

Should an atrial or Junctional automaticity focus become irritable*, it may fire a spontaneous impulse that depolarizes the surrounding tissue, so we can recognize it on _____ as a premature beat.   EKG

But a *very* _____ atrial or Junctional focus may fire   irritable a series of rapid pacing impulses to become the dominant pacemaker, overdrive-suppressing all automaticity centers.

NOTE: Conditions/substances that can make an atrial (usually) or Junctional focus (occasionally) irritable:
- an excess of epinephrine or norepinephrine, the natural substances that stimulate the adrenergic receptors (of foci).
- adrenergic chemicals that mimic this effect.
- substances or conditions that increase the release of epinephrine or norepinephrine.

* Recalling an irritable person who suddenly yelled at you (too much adrenaline, or maybe too much coffee), you will remember that upper level foci can also become "irritable" (same causes) and spontaneously fire a stimulus.

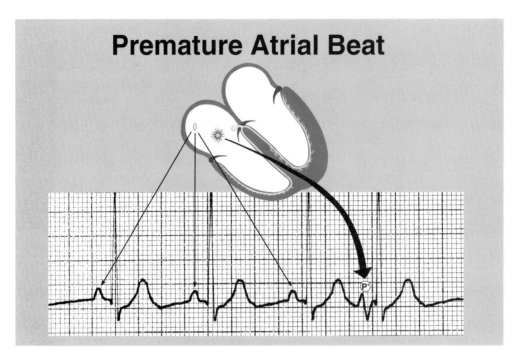

Premature Atrial Beat

A *Premature Atrial Beat* (PAB) originates suddenly in an irritable (see previous page) atrial automaticity focus, and it produces an abnormal P' wave earlier than expected. On EKG, P' (called "P prime") is atrial depolarization by a focus.

A Premature Atrial Beat (PAB) originates in an irritable atrial automaticity focus which spontaneously fires a depolarization stimulus earlier than the normal ___ wave on EKG.

P

But because an atrial focus is the origin of this premature atrial depolarization (not the SA Node), the stimulus produces a premature and unusually shaped P' wave* configuration that does not look like a normal Sinus-generated P _____.

wave

NOTE: On EKG a PAB records as a P'. The P' may be difficult to detect when it's hiding on the peak of a T wave; the giveaway is a too-tall T...taller than the other T waves in the same lead.

NOTE: A PAB also depolarizes the SA Node; that must have some effect...

*Atrial depolarization from a focus near the SA Node produces a generally upright P' wave, whereas foci in the lower atrium depolarize the atria in a "bottom-upwards" (retrograde) fashion to record an inverted P' wave.

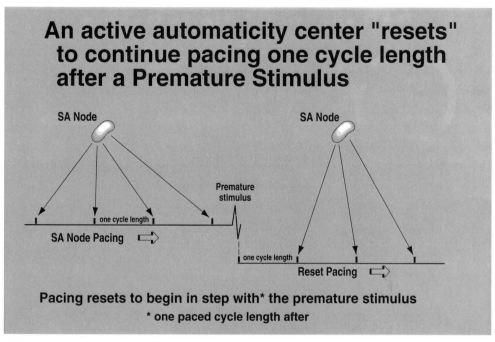

An active automaticity center "resets" to continue pacing one cycle length after a Premature Stimulus

SA Node

SA Node

Premature stimulus

one cycle length

SA Node Pacing

one cycle length

Reset Pacing

Pacing resets to begin in step with* the premature stimulus
* one paced cycle length after

All centers of automaticity **reset**, a characteristic of automaticity. A center of automaticity resets its rhythm when it is depolarized by a premature stimulus, so its pacemaking activity resets in step with the premature beat.

Resetting occurs when the dominant automaticity center (usually the SA Node) is depolarized by a _____ beat, then...

premature

...its pacemaking activity resets in step with the premature stimulus, so that the next pacing stimulus that it generates is one cycle length from the premature _____.

beat
(stimulus)

If the SA Node is depolarized by a premature beat, the SA Node pacemaking is reset so that its regular pacing resumes one cycle length from the _____ stimulus.

premature

NOTE: In order to reset, the dominant (active) center of automaticity must be depolarized by the premature beat. When there is a premature stimulus that does not reach the dominant pacing center, its pacing is not reset.

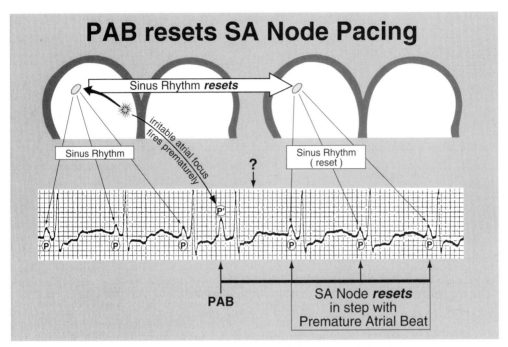

A Premature Atrial Beat from an irritable atrial automaticity focus produces
a too-early depolarization of the atria that depolarizes the SA Node as well.
So the SA Node resets its rhythm in step with the Premature Atrial Beat (P').

NOTE: The P' on EKG is the funny-looking atrial depolarization wave
produced by an automaticity focus. It appears different from all
SA Node-generated P waves in the same EKG lead, but a normal QRS follows.

If a Regular Sinus Rhythm produced by the SA _____ is interrupted   Node
by a spontaneous Premature Atrial Beat (from an atrial automaticity focus),
the SA Node, which lies within the atria, is depolarized as well so...

...the SA Node resets, making the P' is the first beat of its (reset)
_____. The "?" in the illustration marks where the P wave   rhythm
would have occurred, if the SA Node weren't reset.

NOTE: The reset <u>rhythm</u> of the SA Node paces at the same rate (same cycle
length) as before the premature stimulus, but it continues in step with the P'.
The pacing <u>rate</u> of the SA Node before and after the PAB remains the same.

NOTE: In reality, the first cycle after a PAB is a little lengthened due to a
transient (baroreceptor) parasympathetic effect on the SA Node, which resumes
pacing during systole. (Understanding the mechanism is not important.)

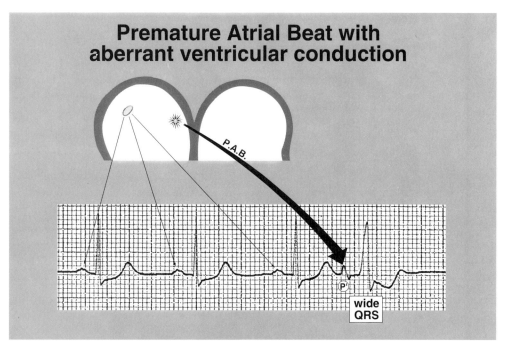

Premature Atrial Beat with aberrant ventricular conduction

P.A.B.

P'

wide QRS

The ventricular conduction system is usually receptive to being depolarized by a Premature Atrial Beat, but one Bundle Branch may not have completely <u>r</u>epolarized when the other is receptive. This *aberrant ventricular conduction* produces a slightly widened QRS (for that premature cycle only).

NOTE: When a Premature Atrial Beat (P') is conducted to the ventricles, the ventricles are also depolarized earlier than usual.

Sometimes a Premature Atrial Beat can produce aberrant ventricular conduction because one of the Bundle Branches is not completely _____ and therefore temporarily   repolarized
refractory to depolarization.

So, depolarization to one ventricle is immediate, while depolarization of the other ventricle is slightly _____.   delayed

The non-simultaneous depolarization of both ventricles records as a slightly _____ QRS complex after the P' on the EKG.   widened
Then, normal ventricular conduction resumes with normal cycles.

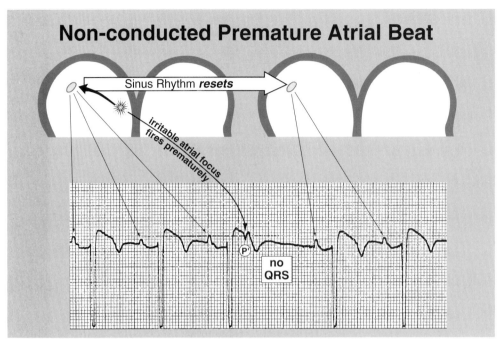

Non-conducted Premature Atrial Beat

Sinus Rhythm *resets*

irritable atrial focus fires prematurely

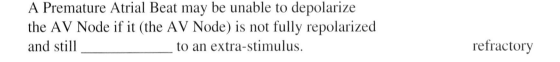

(P')

no
QRS

At times, the AV Node is completely unreceptive to a premature atrial depolarization stimulus because the AV Node is still in the refractory period of its repolarization. This results in a "*non-conducted*" (to the ventricles) Premature Atrial Beat.

A Premature Atrial Beat may be unable to depolarize
the AV Node if it (the AV Node) is not fully repolarized
and still _____ to an extra-stimulus.   refractory

On EKG this records as a too-early, unusual ___ wave   P'
that has no ventricular (QRS-T) response.

NOTE: Warning! Although a "non-conducted" PAB (on EKG, a premature P' without a QRS response) does not depolarize the ventricles, it does depolarize the SA Node, which resets its pacemaking one cycle length from the premature stimulus. The combination of reset pacing plus the missing QRS-T creates a harmless, but dangerous-looking, span of empty baseline...which has the sinister appearance of a "some-kind-of-block." And one day you will have the satisfaction of correcting someone who guessed the wrong diagnosis.

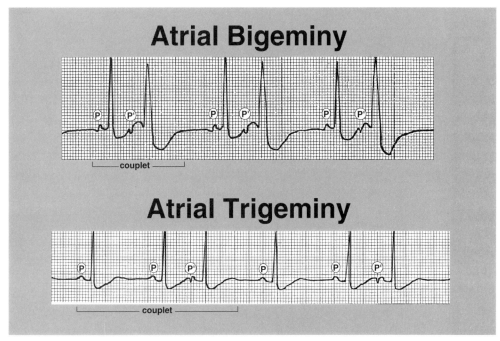

Atrial Bigeminy

couplet

Atrial Trigeminy

couplet

Occasionally, an irritable automaticity focus fires a Premature Atrial Beat (P') at the end of a normal cycle, and repeats this process by coupling a PAB to the end of each successive normal cycle. This is *Atrial Bigeminy.*

NOTE: The cycle containing the premature beat together with the cycle or cycles to which it couples, is called a "couplet."

When an irritable atrial focus repeatedly couples a PAB to the end of each (otherwise normal) cycle, this is a run of _____ Bigeminy*.   Atrial

Sometimes, an irritable atrial focus may prematurely fire after two normal cycles; when this couplet _____ continuously,   repeats it is a run of *Atrial Trigeminy.*

NOTE: With both Atrial Bigeminy and Atrial Trigeminy, each premature stimulus (from the irritable atrial focus) depolarizes the SA Node and resets it, so there is a span of clear baseline between the couplets. So a series (run) of couplet groups called "group beating" is often seen with Atrial Bigeminy, Trigeminy, etc. If you see a premature beat in each couplet, it must be couplets of premature beats. It's that simple! This is mentioned because group beating may occur with a type of AV conduction block to be discussed later (page 171).

*As you may have noticed, there is a slightly widened (aberrant) QRS after each P' in the upper tracing. Aberrant ventricular conduction can occur after any premature atrial (or Junctional) beat.

Practice Tracings

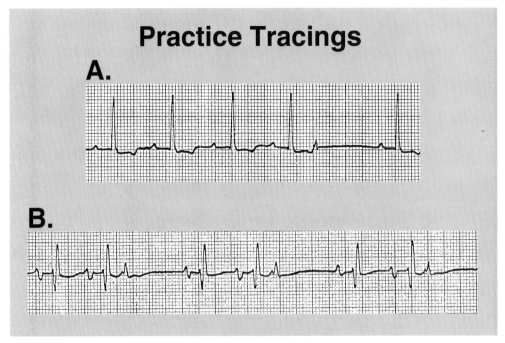

A.

B.

Can you determine what is occurring on each of these practice EKG tracings?

Tracing A: This tracing is from a medical student who had a few cups of coffee in order to study late. She stopped by the Emergency Room because her pulse seemed irregular.

    The intern on duty thought that the tracing showed "intermittent complete AV Block" and was about to call the attending physician (at 4:00 AM) to schedule an emergency artificial pacemaker implantation. Explain the EKG strip to the intern, using only what you have learned so far (before he wakes the attending physician and discovers the real meaning of "irritable") .

Tracing B: This transmitted telemetry tracing is from a known drug abuser who took a large quantity of amphetamines before his ride to the hospital.

    Someone in the ambulance suggested what sounded like "Winky bok block", when the telemetry was received. Utilizing only what you have read and understood so far in this book, you recognize a combination of things that you have just learned. You do notice that in each grouping only two of the P waves are identical. Slowly analyze what you see, so you can explain it to others.

NOTE: Carefully examine each tracing and contemplate its written information. The answers will appear as you continue in the book...somewhere.

Premature Junctional Beat

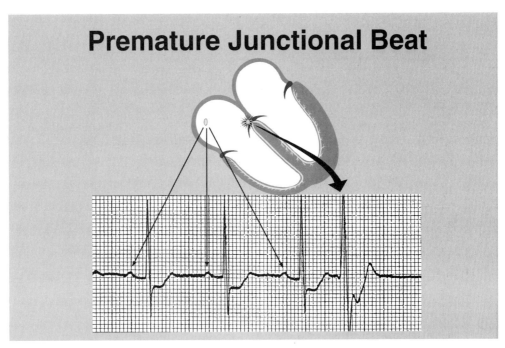

A *Premature Junctional Beat* (PJB) occurs when an irritable automaticity focus in the AV Junction suddenly fires a premature stimulus that is conducted to, and depolarizes, the ventricles (and sometimes the atria).

When an irritable focus (see page 119) in the AV Junction spontaneously fires a stimulus, this produces a Premature
_____ Beat on EKG.   Junctional

NOTE: When heart tissue depolarizes, it immediately repolarizes, and during repolarization that tissue is refractory to another stimulus (premature stimulus). As the ventricles repolarize, one Bundle Branch may repolarize faster than the other. So the too-early depolarization from a PJB may conduct through one Bundle Branch, but the impulse is temporarily blocked in the other, still refractory, Bundle Branch (usually the right). So, instead of depolarizing simultaneously, one ventricle depolarizes slightly before the other, producing a slightly widened QRS complex typical of a Premature Junctional Beat with *aberrant ventricular conduction.*

If you see a premature QRS complex that is slightly widened, you should consider that it may be due to a Premature Junctional (or Premature Atrial) Beat with _____ ventricular conduction.   aberrant

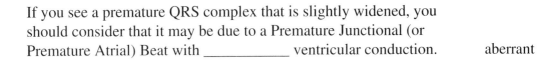

Previous page answers: A. Non-conducted PAB. B. Atrial Trigeminy with non-conducted PAB.

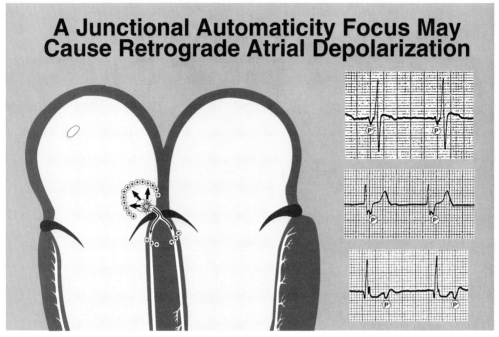

A Junctional Automaticity Focus May Cause Retrograde Atrial Depolarization

A Premature Junctional Beat originates in an irritable Junctional focus within the AV Node. We expect such a premature stimulus to conduct to the ventricles, but it may also depolarize the atria in a bottom-up "retrograde" fashion that records as an *inverted* P' wave on EKG.

The premature P' wave produced by _____ atrial depolarization is inverted (i.e., opposite the QRS on EKG).

retrograde

If a PJB produces retrograde atrial depolarization, it can record an _____ P' wave on EKG immediately before the premature QRS.

inverted

Sometimes an inverted ___ wave associated with a PJB follows the QRS. Occasionally the P' disappears within the QRS when atrial and ventricular depolarization occur simultaneously (not shown in illustration).

P'

NOTE: Retrograde atrial depolarization from a PJB usually depolarizes the SA Node as well. So the SA Node resets its pacing in step with the retrograde *atrial* depolarization.

128

(AV) Junctional Bigeminy

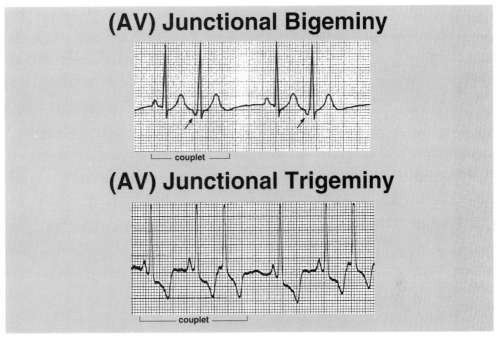

couplet

(AV) Junctional Trigeminy

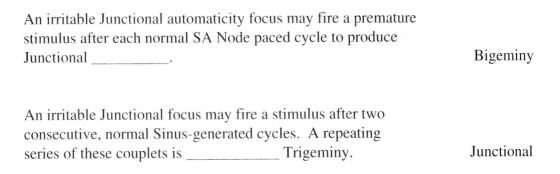

couplet

An irritable automaticity focus in the AV Junction may initiate a Premature Junctional Beat after each normal (SA Node-generated) cycle. This is *Junctional Bigeminy*. When a PJB is coupled with two consecutive, normal cycles in a continuous series of these couplets, this is *Junctional Trigeminy*.

An irritable Junctional automaticity focus may fire a premature stimulus after each normal SA Node paced cycle to produce Junctional _____.

Bigeminy

An irritable Junctional focus may fire a stimulus after two consecutive, normal Sinus-generated cycles. A repeating series of these couplets is _____ Trigeminy.

Junctional

NOTE: Don't forget that on EKG you may see an inverted (retrograde) P' wave (arrows in upper tracing) with every PJB in either Junctional Bigeminy or Trigeminy. Also, the SA Node will reset its pacing with each retrograde atrial depolarization; this can produce alarming gaps of empty baseline between couplets.

A <u>ventricular</u> focus can be made irritable by:

Low O$_2$ Airway obstruction
Absence of air
      (near-drowning or suffocation)
Air with poor O2 content
Minimal oxygenation in lungs
      (pulmonary embolus or pneumothorax)
Reduced cardiac output
      (hypovolemic or cardiogenic shock)
Poor to absent coronary blood supply
      (coronary insufficiency or infarction)

Low K$^+$ Reduced serum potassium ("hypokalemia")

**. . . and to a lesser degree, epinephrine-like substances
(β_1 adrenergic stimulants) and stretch.**

A *ventricular focus* (or sometimes a focus above the ventricles) may become **irritable** from under-oxygenation ("hypoxia") caused by a variety of circumstances and conditions. Ventricular foci are more sensitive to low oxygen than are atrial or Junctional foci.

Poor oxygenation (hypoxia) can make a ventricular automaticity _____ become irritable and fire a spontaneous impulse,   focus
producing a premature beat on EKG.

A very irritable ventricular automaticity focus may be so excessively provoked by hypoxia or "ischemia" (diminished blood supply) that it suddenly fires a series of rapid impulses, overdrive-suppressing the _____ sinus rhythm...   normal
...so it becomes the dominant pacemaker with a rapid rate.

NOTE: If you study the illustration for a moment, you will quickly realize that there are a multitude of mechanisms that can reduce the oxygen supply to these sensitive ventricular automaticity foci, and not all of these mechanisms are illustrated. In a clinical setting, most (but not all) "deadly" emergency ventricular tachycardias are due to coronary insufficiency or infarction.

NOTE: Cocaine is known to make atrial and Junctional foci irritable, but it has more sinister effects. Cocaine causes coronary spasm, making ventricular foci hypoxic AND very irritable; dangerous ventricular arrhythmias may ensue.

130

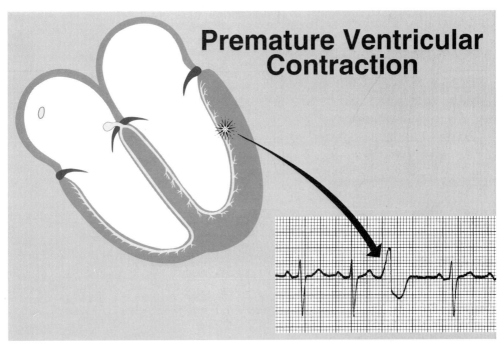

Premature Ventricular Contraction

A premature ventricular beat is called a *Premature Ventricular Contraction* (PVC*). It originates suddenly in an irritable automaticity focus in a ventricle and produces a giant ventricular complex on EKG.

An irritable (please, quickly review the previous page) ventricular focus may suddenly fire a stimulus and produce a _____ Ventricular Complex (PVC) on EKG.   Premature

NOTE: PVC's occur early in the cycle. Easily recognized by their great width and enormous amplitude (height and depth), they are usually opposite the polarity of the normal QRS's (e.g. if QRS's are upward, PVC's are mainly downward).

The most likely reason for a ventricular automaticity focus to become irritable is under-_____ (hypoxia).   oxygenation

NOTE: PVC denotes a ventricular "contraction." When you see a PVC, remember that this represents a (premature) ventricular contraction, and a premature pulse beat, albeit weaker than normal (the ventricles are not completely filled).

* PVC may stand for Premature Ventricular "Contraction" or "Complex." The issue remains unresolved.

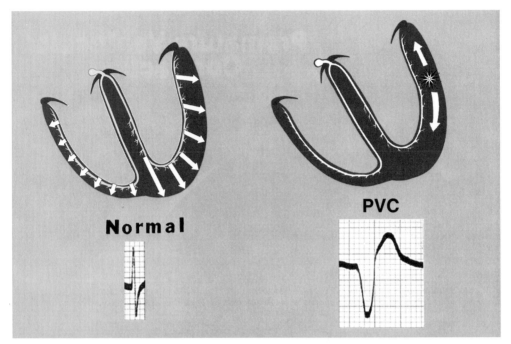

Normal   PVC

The PVC originates in an automaticity focus (in a Purkinje fiber) within the ventricular conduction system, somewhere in the wall of a ventricle. Thus one area of the ventricular wall begins to depolarize before the rest of the ventricle and long before the other ventricle depolarizes.

NOTE: After a normal, Sinus-generated depolarization stimulus has passed through the AV Node, the stimulus is quickly transmitted to the entire endocardial lining of both ventricles at once. This simultaneous depolarization of both ventricles produces a nice, slender QRS complex on EKG.

NOTE: When an irritable ventricular automaticity focus suddenly fires an impulse, the region of ventricular wall where it is located depolarizes before the rest of the ventricle, and then the depolarization wave creeps to the other ventricle, which then depolarizes...producing an enormously wide ventricular complex.

NOTE: Normally, ventricular depolarization passes through the entire thickness of both ventricles at once. Left ventricular depolarization in the leftward direction tends to be counterbalanced by the simultaneous right ventricular depolarization in the opposite direction. This minimizes the amplitude of the QRS waves on EKG. But depolarization originating in a remote ventricular focus (as with a PVC) gradually spreads without simultaneous opposition from other areas, and in its slow course, produces (unopposed) deflections of immense amplitude.

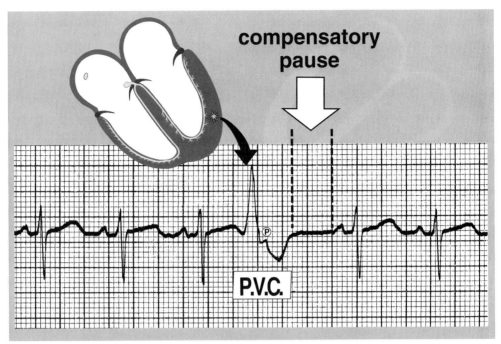

The PVC is an enormous ventricular complex that is much wider, taller, and deeper than a normal QRS. There is a pause after the PVC, but it is <u>not</u> caused by resetting of the SA Node, in fact, sometimes you can see the punctual, but ineffective P wave within the PVC (see P in illustration).

The PVC is a gigantic ventricular complex that jumps out at you from the EKG, warning you that there is a ventricular focus that is irritable because of _____.   hypoxia

The PVC depolarizes the _____, but not the SA Node,   ventricles
so the SA Node discharges on schedule. In fact by measuring P-P cycles, you can often locate the punctual P wave within a PVC.

But that timely P wave occurs while the ventricles are still refractory (from the PVC) and not fully _____.   repolarized
When this normal stimulus arrives, they can't depolarize...

...so there is a _____ as the ventricles finish repolarizing   pause*
to make them receptive to the next Sinus-generated cycle.

NOTE: *Interpolated PVC's* are rare, but are somehow sandwiched between the beats of a normal rhythm, producing no pause and no rhythm disturbance.

* The pause, sometimes called a "compensatory" pause, doesn't "compensate" for anything.

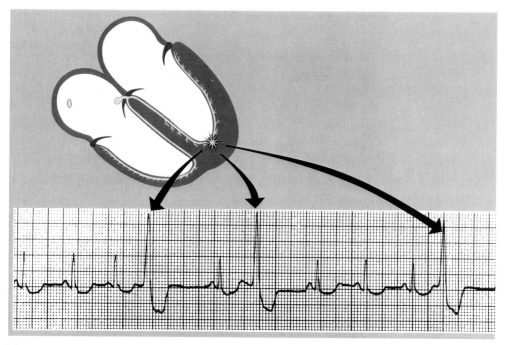

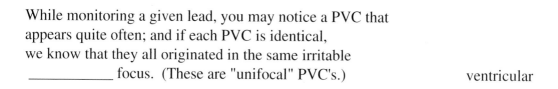

Numerous PVC's may emanate from the same ventricular focus, warning that the focus is very irritable because of its poor state of oxygenation. Six or more PVC's per minute is considered pathological.

While monitoring a given lead, you may notice a PVC that
appears quite often; and if each PVC is identical,
we know that they all originated in the same irritable
_____ focus. (These are "unifocal" PVC's.)   ventricular

The presence of many unifocal PVC's indicates poor oxygenation
of a ventricular focus – usually because the heart's own coronary
blood supply is diminished. Remember, ___ PVC's per minute   Six (6)
is pathological. Don't ignore this patient!

NOTE: There are situations when the coronary blood flow is adequate,
but the blood is poorly oxygenated (e.g., drowning, pulmonary embolus,
tracheal obstruction, etc.). When a highly irritable ventricular focus is
warning you with multiple PVC's...you must respond! Low serum potassium,
as well as certain chemicals and medications, can also irritate a ventricular
focus. In addition, adrenergic stimulants like epinephrine can aggravate the
situation.

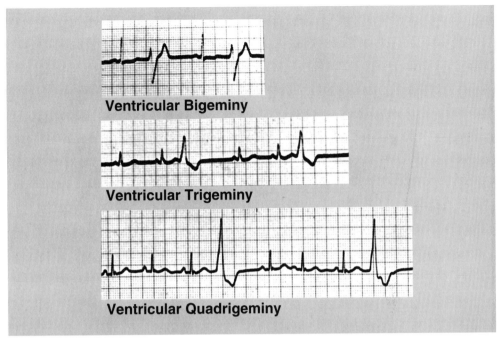

Ventricular Bigeminy

Ventricular Trigeminy

Ventricular Quadrigeminy

A very irritable ventricular automaticity focus may fire a stimulus that couples with one or more normal cycles to produce *Ventricular Bigeminy,* or *Ventricular Trigeminy,* etc.

NOTE: Keep in mind our conventional 6 PVC's per minute, which is pathological. A continuous run of any of these couplet patterns quickly exceeds that criterion and indicates that a very irritable focus is hypoxic and calling for help.

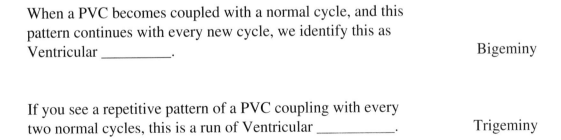

When a PVC becomes coupled with a normal cycle, and this pattern continues with every new cycle, we identify this as Ventricular _____.

Bigeminy

If you see a repetitive pattern of a PVC coupling with every two normal cycles, this is a run of Ventricular _____.

Trigeminy

NOTE: Ventricular automaticity foci are the heart's hypoxia early warning system. Respond!

Ventricular Parasystole

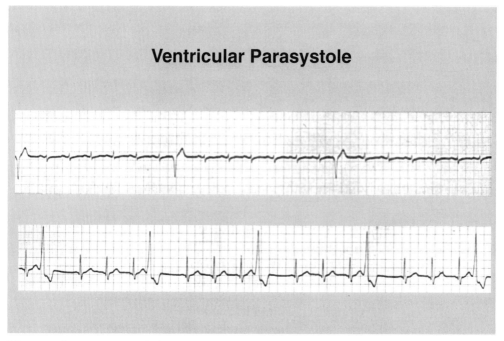

Ventricular Parasystole is produced by a ventricular focus that suffers from entrance block, so the focus is insensitive to overdrive suppression. It continues to pace at its inherent rate, and its ventricular complexes poke through the dominant Sinus Rhythm.

NOTE: "Entrance Block" is a condition (usually due to hypoxia) that insulates ("protects") an automaticity focus from being depolarized by incoming stimuli, thereby preventing overdrive suppression. However, an entrance-blocked focus can still successfully deliver its own pacing stimuli.

NOTE: Sometimes a ventricular automaticity focus has entrance block, which prevents its depolarization by outside sources. Without overdrive suppression, it paces at its inherent rate. The result is a dual rhythm with pacing from two sources, the SA Node and the ventricular focus.

When you see PVC's that appear to be coupled to a long series of normal cycles, you should suspect Ventricular _____.   Parasystole

NOTE: Because this represents two unrelated, independent rhythms (from two different pacing locations), the interval between the normal cycle and the large ventricular complex is not consistent. Occasionally a large ventricular complex may fail to appear because the ventricular focus happens to discharge during the refractory period of the (Sinus-paced) ventricles.

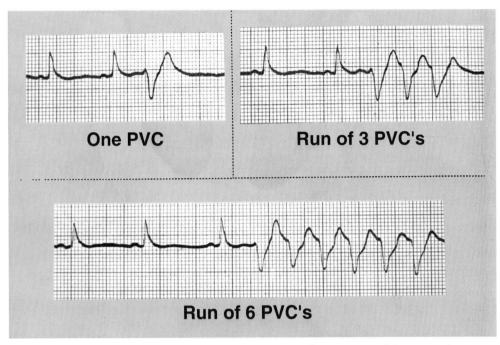

One PVC

Run of 3 PVC's

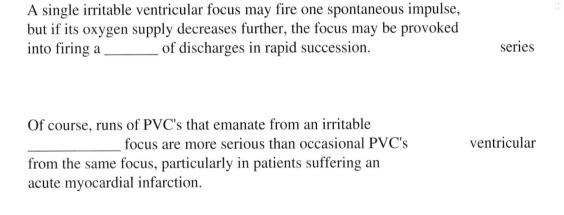

Run of 6 PVC's

An irritable ventricular automaticity focus may fire once or, if extremely irritable (under-oxygenated), it may fire a series of rapid impulses to produce a run of PVC's.

A single irritable ventricular focus may fire one spontaneous impulse, but if its oxygen supply decreases further, the focus may be provoked into firing a _____ of discharges in rapid succession.   series

Of course, runs of PVC's that emanate from an irritable _____ focus are more serious than occasional PVC's   ventricular from the same focus, particularly in patients suffering an acute myocardial infarction.

NOTE: A run of three or more PVC's in rapid succession is called a run of *Ventricular Tachycardia* (VT). Two of the examples in the above illustration are VT. If a run of VT lasts longer than 30 seconds, it is called "sustained" VT.

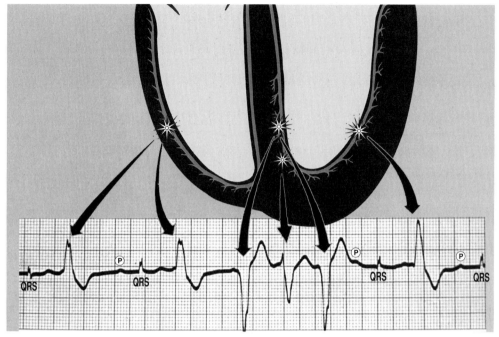

Severe cardiac hypoxia can cause *Multifocal* PVC's — a desperation measure produced by multiple, exceptionally irritable (hypoxic), ventricular automaticity foci. Each focus produces its own unique, identifiable PVC every time it fires.

In a given lead, PVC's originating in a specific ventricular
focus all appear the _____.   same

NOTE: Severe cardiac hypoxia can cause the appearance of numerous multifocal PVC's. This is indeed dangerous and requires immediate intervention. Because a single irritable ventricular focus can suddenly fire a series of rapid discharges to produce a dangerous tachy-arrhythmia (e.g., Ventricular Tachycardia), the presence of numerous multifocal PVC's means that a number of extremely irritable foci are discharging, and trouble is imminent. The chance of developing a dangerous or even deadly arrhythmia (e.g., Ventricular Fibrillation) under these dire circumstances is obviously enhanced. With infarction patients, this is an alarm of crisis proportions!

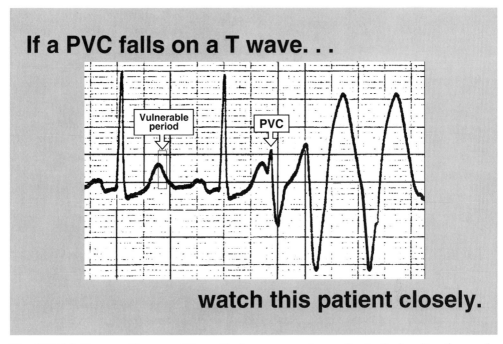

If a PVC falls on a T wave. . .

Vulnerable period

PVC

watch this patient closely.

If a PVC falls on a T wave (*R on T phenomenon*), particularly in situations of hypoxia or low serum potassium, it occurs during a "vulnerable period" and dangerous arrhythmias may result. See in the illustration, how a PVC hits the second T wave directly in its vulnerable period...and see what happens.

PVC's are, of course, premature and usually
occur just after the ___ wave of a normal cycle.   T

When a PVC falls on the peak of a T wave or on the initial part
of its downslope, it catches the ventricles during a vulnerable period,
particularly in the presence of _____ (often caused by cardiac   hypoxia
ischemia from a narrowed coronary artery) or in the presence
of low potassium.

NOTE: With an ischemic myocardium, the vulnerable period extends
beyond the T wave, so that a PVC falling just after the T wave
may occur during this (extended) vulnerable period.

NOTE: Although this is a well known warning sign, "R on T" is often noted
after the fact, during the review of an EKG strip from a patient who suffered a
dangerous or deadly arrhythmia. By being cautious and vigilant, you may
prevent a problem like this from occurring.

PRACTICE TRACING

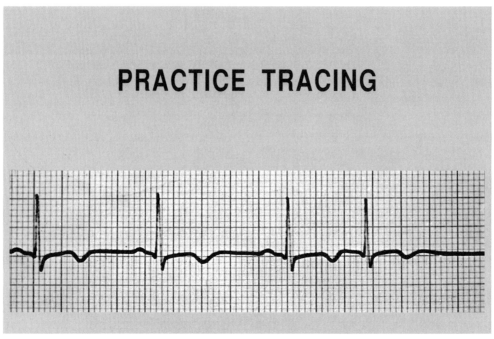

The discerning eye of a coronary care nurse detected a beat that appeared a little too early on the EKG strip taken from a patient's monitor. Let's determine the location of the irritable focus that produced the premature beat.

The last QRS complex in the strip catches your eye because it occurs prematurely, and it is not preceded by a ___ wave.   P

The last QRS complex looks the same as the other QRS's, so we know that, although premature, the last QRS resulted from depolarization that passed (in a normal fashion) down the ventricular conduction system. Therefore, it is <u>not</u> from a _____ focus.   ventricular

Carefully examining the EKG strip, we don't see a P' (with a little baseline) before the premature QRS, so we know that the QRS did not emanate from an atrial focus. Therefore the irritable automaticity focus that produced the premature QRS must be in the ___ _____.   AV Junction

NOTE: Sure you understand this, but it probably would be a good idea to take a minute and review some of the subtle characteristics of premature beats. I'll wait.

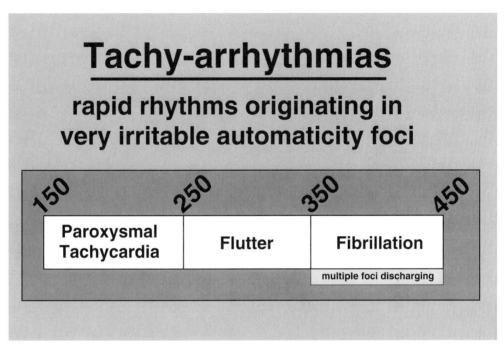

Tachy-arrhythmias

rapid rhythms originating in very irritable automaticity foci

150	250	350	450
Paroxysmal Tachycardia	**Flutter**	**Fibrillation**	
		multiple foci discharging	

A *Tachy-arrhythmia* originates in a very irritable focus that paces rapidly. Sometimes more than one active focus is generating pacing stimuli at once.

NOTE: Tachy-arrhythmia ("rapid arrhythmia"), hyphenated for recognition purposes, is not usually hyphenated, so henceforth I'll omit the hyphen.

The range of rates of the tachyarrhythmias are:

Paroxysmal Tachycardia...... _____ to _____ /minute.   150 to 250

Flutter................................. _____ to _____ /minute.   250 to 350

Fibrillation........................... _____ to _____ /minute.   350 to 450

NOTE: A tachyarrhythmia is easily recognized by rate alone, but the specific diagnosis requires that we identify the origin, that is, we must determine the location of the irritable automaticity focus (atrial, Junctional, or ventricular). You already have a solid understanding* of normal conduction in the heart, so we merely need to get up to speed (pun intended) in learning the behavior of very irritable automaticity foci, and how they record on EKG.

* "Understanding is a kind of ecstacy."   Carl Sagan (from *Broca's Brain*).

Paroxysmal (sudden) Tachycardia
- a very irritable automaticity focus suddenly paces rapidly:

- **Paroxysmal Atrial Tachycardia**
- **Paroxysmal Junctional Tachycardia**
- **Paroxysmal Ventricular Tachycardia**

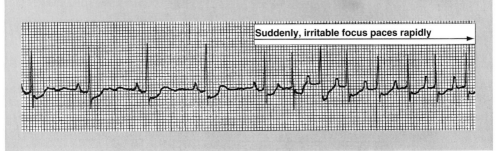

Suddenly, irritable focus paces rapidly

Paroxysmal ("sudden") *Tachycardia* ("rapid heart rate") indicates rapid pacing (150 to 250/ minute) by a <u>very</u> irritable automaticity focus. Once we recognize a paroxysmal tachycardia, we need only identify the focus (atrial, Junctional, or ventricular) of its origin.

The medical term for rapid heart rate is _____.   tachycardia

Paroxysmal means _____.   sudden

NOTE: Paroxysmal Tachycardia arises <u>suddenly</u> from a very irritable automaticity focus. Generally speaking, stimulants like epinephrine make higher level foci irritable, whereas more threatening physiological conditions like hypoxia (or low potassium) make ventricular foci irritable. There is some overlap, however. In addition, a single premature stimulus from another focus can provoke an irritable focus into a run of Paroxysmal Tachycardia.

In contrast, Sinus Tachycardia is the SA Node's <u>gradual</u> response to exercise, excitement, etc. Although the SA Node's rate of pacing may become quite rapid, Sinus Tachycardia is neither sudden nor does it originate in an automaticity focus, so by definition, this is NOT a _____ Tachycardia.   Paroxysmal

142

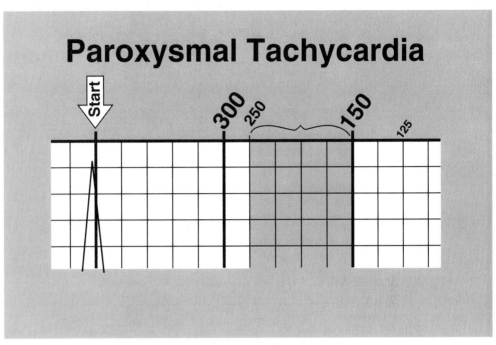

The rate range of the paroxysmal tachycardias is 150* to 250 per minute, so they are easy to recognize. Locating the causative irritable focus (atrial, Junctional, or ventricular) gives us the diagnosis.

When calculating rate, we find an R wave that peaks on a heavy black "start" line. The next three heavy black lines are called "300, 150, ____."

100

The fine line immediately to the right of the heavy black "300" line is the thin "250" line. Therefore, if an R wave falls on the "start" line (see illustration) the next R wave will fall within the shaded area during paroxysmal _____.

tachycardia

You can instantly recognize a paroxysmal tachycardia by noting the rate range of _____ to 250 per minute. Now you have to determine at which of three levels there is a very irritable automaticity focus causing the tachycardia. Easy enough!

150

* Some authors now set the lower rate limit of Paroxysmal Tachycardia at 125/ minute.

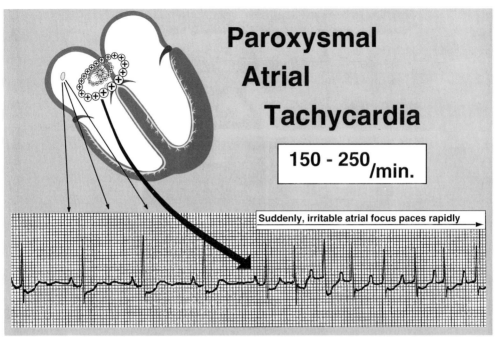

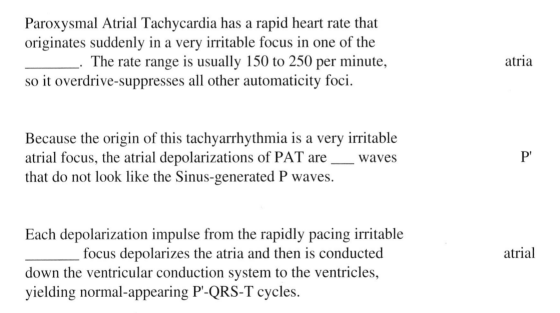

Paroxysmal Atrial Tachycardia (PAT) is caused by the sudden, rapid firing of a very irritable* atrial automaticity focus. You may see the beginning of this arrhythmia only occasionally, so become familiar with its general appearance.

Paroxysmal Atrial Tachycardia has a rapid heart rate that originates suddenly in a very irritable focus in one of the _____. The rate range is usually 150 to 250 per minute, so it overdrive-suppresses all other automaticity foci.

atria

Because the origin of this tachyarrhythmia is a very irritable atrial focus, the atrial depolarizations of PAT are ___ waves that do not look like the Sinus-generated P waves.

P'

Each depolarization impulse from the rapidly pacing irritable _____ focus depolarizes the atria and then is conducted down the ventricular conduction system to the ventricles, yielding normal-appearing P'-QRS-T cycles.

atrial

NOTE: A premature stimulus from another focus may set off a run of PAT.

* Quickly review page 119.

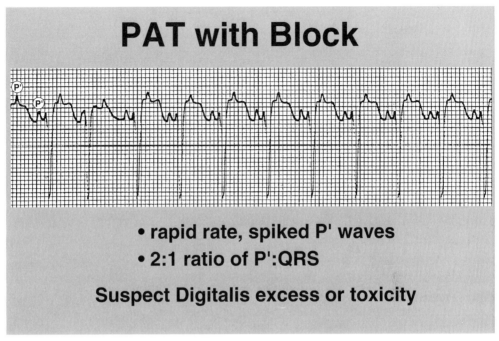

PAT with Block

- **rapid rate, spiked P' waves**
- **2:1 ratio of P':QRS**

Suspect Digitalis excess or toxicity

In *Paroxysmal Atrial Tachycardia with block* there is more than one P' wave spike for every QRS response. Suspect digitalis excess or even toxicity; atrial foci are very sensitive to the irritating effects of digitalis preparations.

NOTE: Excess digitalis can provoke an atrial focus into such an irritable state that it suddenly paces rapidly. At the same time, digitalis markedly slows conduction in the AV Node, so that only every second stimulus conducts to the ventricles (every-other atrial stimulus is blocked in the AV Node).

PAT with block is a tachyarrhythmia that has two P' waves for each QRS response on EKG, because the ___ _____ blocks the conduction of every-other atrial stimulus.   AV Node

PAT with block is usually a sign of _____ excess or toxicity,   digitalis
particularly if the patient has a low serum potassium, so careful
administration of intravenous potassium is usually therapeutic.

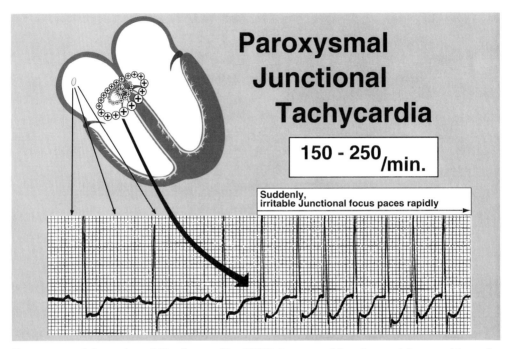

Paroxysmal Junctional Tachycardia

150 - 250/min.

Suddenly, irritable Junctional focus paces rapidly

Paroxysmal Junctional Tachycardia (PJT) is caused by the sudden rapid pacing of a very irritable automaticity focus in the AV Junction. The Junctional focus may suddenly initiate tachycardia pacing because of marked irritability induced by stimulants and/or by a premature beat from another focus.

Paroxysmal Junctional Tachycardia is due to a very irritable* focus
in the AV Junction that paces at the rate of _____ to 250 per minute.   150

NOTE: A rapidly pacing (irritable) Junctional focus *may* also depolarize the atria from below in retrograde fashion to record:
- an inverted P' immediately before each QRS, or   (see illustration
- an inverted P' after each QRS, or   page 128)
- an inverted P' buried within each QRS (difficult to detect).

NOTE: Each stimulus from a rapidly pacing (irritable) Junctional focus may occur at a time in the cycle when the Left Bundle Branch has fully repolarized (i.e. recovered from its refractory period), but the Right Bundle Branch is still refractory (in some patients, the reverse occurs). As a result, this *aberrant ventricular conduction* depolarizes the left ventricle before the right, to produce somewhat widened QRS's during the tachycardia.

*One more look at page 119, and I'll never bother you again.

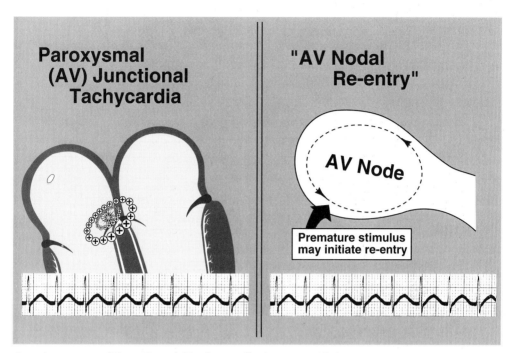

Another type of Junctional Tachycardia is *AV Nodal Reentry* Tachycardia* (AVNRT). In theory, a continuous reentry circuit develops within the AV Node (sometimes including the lower atria) and rapidly paces the atria and ventricles.

NOTE: A theoretical reentry circuit may continuously circle in the AV Junctional region, giving off a depolarization stimulus to the atria and to the ventricles with each pass in the circuit. This is "circus reentry", an aptly named tachycardia that looks suspiciously like PJT.

NOTE: In AVNRT, each pacing stimulus first records from an origin near the coronary sinus – an area loaded with automaticity foci. In addition, although catheter ablation of that area is currently used to eliminate this tachycardia (very suggestive of focal automaticity pacing), dogmatic loyalty to in this theoretical reentry model persists. It is also interesting that AVNRT often records on EKG with inverted P' waves and sometimes with widened QRS's (aberrant ventricular conduction). The jury is still out.

*Pronounced "ree-EN-tree".

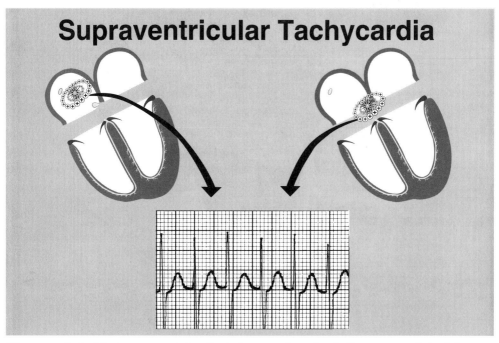

Supraventricular Tachycardia

The very irritable* automaticity foci that produce both Paroxysmal Atrial Tachycardia and Paroxysmal Junctional Tachycardia originate above the ventricles, so they are known as *Paroxysmal Supraventricular Tachycardia.*

Supraventricular Tachycardia (the word "paroxysmal" is often omitted) is a general term, which includes both PAT and _____.   PJT

The term "supraventricular" imparts the understanding that all atrial foci and all Junctional foci are above the _____.   ventricles

NOTE: Paroxysmal Atrial Tachycardia may be so rapid that the P' waves run into the preceding T waves to become indistinguishable. This can make differentiation between PAT and PJT very difficult. But since treatment for both is very similar, the umbrella term Supraventricular Tachycardia (SVT) suffices, and further distinction between the two is unnecessary. Certain conditions may widen the QRS's in SVT, so it may then resemble Ventricular Tachycardia (next page).

*Usually an atrial or Junctional focus is made irritable by adrenergic stimulants, but a focus may be further provoked into tachycardia pacing by a premature stimulus from another irritable focus.

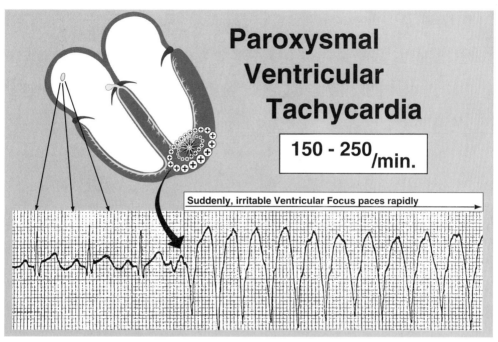

Paroxysmal Ventricular Tachycardia

150 - 250/min.

Suddenly, irritable Ventricular Focus paces rapidly

Paroxysmal Ventricular Tachycardia (PVT or VT)* is produced by a very irritable ventricular automaticity focus that suddenly paces in the 150 to 250 per minute range. It has a characteristic pattern of enormous, consecutive PVC-like complexes. Please conscientiously review page 130 now.

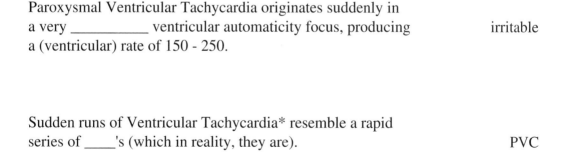

Paroxysmal Ventricular Tachycardia originates suddenly in a very _____ ventricular automaticity focus, producing a (ventricular) rate of 150 - 250.

irritable

Sudden runs of Ventricular Tachycardia* resemble a rapid series of ____'s (which in reality, they are).

PVC

NOTE: During Ventricular Tachycardia, the SA Node still paces the atria, but the large dramatic ventricular complexes hide the individual P waves that can be seen only occasionally. So there is independent pacing of the atria and the ventricles...a type of *AV dissociation*.

* The "Paroxysmal" is often left off, so "Ventricular Tachycardia" and "VT" are used commonly.

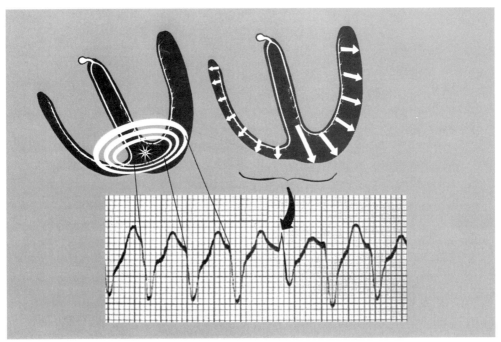

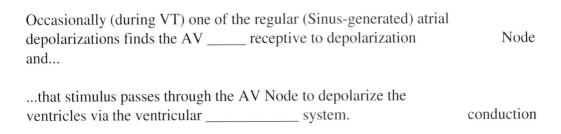

During Ventricular Tachycardia, the SA Node continues to pace the atria (AV dissociation), but only an occasional atrial depolarization catches the AV Node in a receptive state, and then this depolarization stimulus conducts to the ventricles.

Occasionally (during VT) one of the regular (Sinus-generated) atrial depolarizations finds the AV _____ receptive to depolarization and...   Node

...that stimulus passes through the AV Node to depolarize the ventricles via the ventricular _____ system.   conduction

NOTE: On occasion during VT, a (Sinus-generated) depolarization stimulus from the atria finds the entire ventricular conduction system receptive to depolarization and produces a normal appearing QRS (*capture beat*) in the midst of the ventricular tachycardia. More commonly during VT, an atrial depolarization finds a receptive AV Node, but ventricular depolarization only proceeds so far before it meets ventricular depolarization progressing from the ventricular focus. This produces a *fusion beat,* which is a blending on EKG of a normal QRS with a PVC-like complex (see illustration). The presence of "captures" or "fusions" confirms the diagnosis of Ventricular Tachycardia, because they could not occur with a SVT.

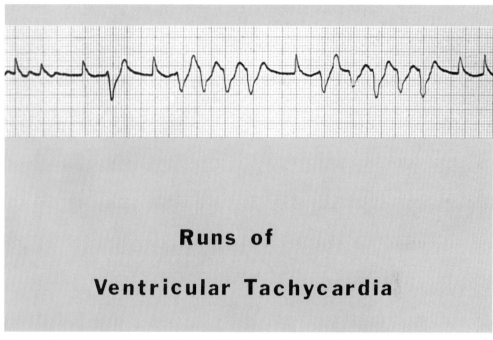

Runs of

Ventricular Tachycardia

Runs of (Paroxysmal) Ventricular Tachycardia may signify coronary insufficiency (ischemia) or other causes of cardiac hypoxia what make a ventricular automaticity focus very irritable.

Ventricular Tachycardia appears like a run of _____'s.   PVC

This is a serious, pathological condition, which often
indicates coronary _____, causing poor   insufficiency
oxygenation of the heart (other causes of cardiac hypoxia
are obviously possible; see page 130).

NOTE: This rapid ventricular rate suddenly erupts from an irritable (hypoxic) ventricular focus. The rapid rate is too fast for the heart to function effectively, particularly in the elderly with compromised coronaries. It should be treated quickly (but cautiously) in patients with a myocardial infarction.

CAUTION: A rapid (Junctional or atrial) Supraventricular Tachycardia with aberrant conduction can produce a tachycardia with widened QRS's that can mimic VT. Also, pre-existing Bundle Branch Block with SVT will widen the QRS complexes to give the same impression . NEVER give medications for SVT to a patient with VT.

Distinguishing
Wide QRS complex SVT from Ventricular Tachycardia

Helpful Clues	Wide QRS complex SVT	Ventricular Tachycardia
Patient with coronary disease or infarction	uncommon	very common
QRS width (duration)	less than .14 sec.	greater than .14 sec.
AV dissociation showing captures or fusions	rare	yes
Axis: Extreme R.A.D.	rare	yes
Q wave in Lead V_6	rare	yes

A few clues and good judgement can help you distinguish between VT and SVT (with aberrant ventricular conduction). Begin with the history, and get a 12 lead EKG.

The patient with VT is most likely elderly and suffering from diminished coronary blood _____, reducing the oxygen supply to his (or her) ventricular foci.   flow

Signs of AV dissociation (e.g., presence of fusions or captures, a Q in V_6, or Extreme R.A.D. (-90° to -180°) is characteristic of ___.   VT

NOTE: If the QRS complex can be measured with accuracy, the QRS in SVT, even if widened by aberrant ventricular conduction, is usually .14 sec. or less in duration. However the ventricular complexes in VT are very wide, .14 sec. or greater. There are many sophisticated methods for distinguishing VT from SVT with aberrancy, but probably the most reliable to date is in:

Brugada et al: The Differential Diagnosis of a Regular Tachycardia with a Wide QRS Complex on the 12 Lead ECG. PACE 1994; Vol.17: 1515-1524.

Torsades de Pointes

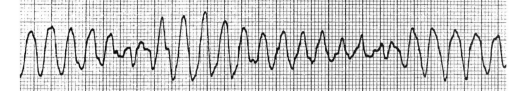

outline looks like a party streamer

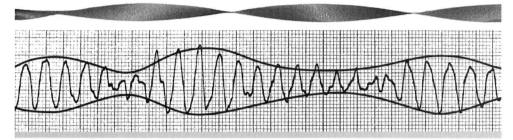

Torsades de Pointes is a peculiar form of (very) rapid ventricular rhythm caused by low potassium, medications (those that block potassium channels), or congenital abnormalities (e.g., Long QT Syndrome) that lengthen the QT interval. The rate is a variable 250 to 350 per minute, in brief episodes.

Quinidine toxicity may cause, p. 297.

NOTE: Torsades de Pointes means "twisting of points" which refers to the series of ventricular complexes that are upward-pointing then downward-pointing complexes in a repeating continuity. In 1966 Dr. F. Dessertenne presented the first scientific description of this arrhythmia. He theorized that it was caused by two competitive, irritable ventricular foci – an explanation that still seems quite plausible.

The rate of this arrhythmia is 250 to ____ per minute, but fortunately it occurs only in brief bursts, for at that rate, there is no effective ventricular pumping.   350

NOTE: The amplitude of each successive complex gradually increases and then gradually decreases, so when viewed as a whole, the general outline or silhouette of the tracing looks like a series of end-to-end spindle shapes. Some say the tracing outline resembles a twisting, party streamer. Untreated, it can be deadly.

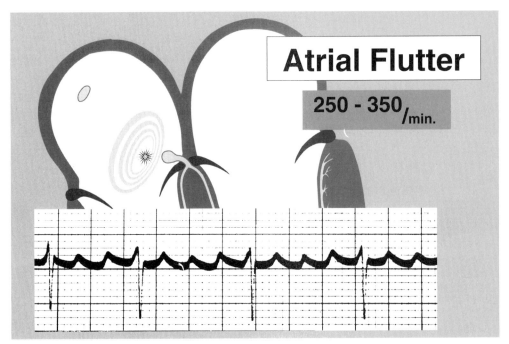

Atrial Flutter

250 - 350 /min.

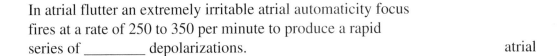

Atrial Flutter originates in an atrial automaticity focus. The atrial depolarization waves, which some call "flutter waves" occur in rapid succession and each is identical to the next.

In atrial flutter an extremely irritable atrial automaticity focus fires at a rate of 250 to 350 per minute to produce a rapid series of _____ depolarizations.   atrial

NOTE: Atrial flutter is characterized by a series of identical "flutter" waves in rapid back-to-back succession. Because the waves are identical, they are described as having the appearance of the teeth of a saw or a "saw tooth" baseline. The baseline appears to vanish between atrial depolarizations; rather, there is only a rapid succession of back-to-back flutter waves. Turn back to PAT with block to make sure that you recognize the difference.

NOTE: The AV Node has an extended refractory period with each cycle that acts as a filter to limit the number of depolarizations that conduct to the ventricles. In this way very rapid atrial rates will not drive the ventricles at the same excessive rate; perhaps only one of two (or commonly, one of three, as above) atrial depolarizations reaches the ventricles in Atrial Flutter.

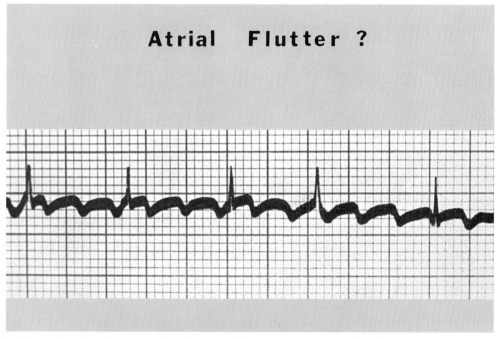

Atrial Flutter ?

This tracing looks somewhat like atrial flutter, but to make it more a more classical, recognizable pattern you have to turn it upside-down.

When in doubt about atrial flutter, inverting the _____ tracing may be helpful.

EKG

NOTE: The diagnosis of atrial flutter is usually made on the basis of its unmistakable appearance on EKG. Because there is only one atrial focus pacing, each "P' wave" (called a *flutter* wave) looks identical to all the others. Some believe that this is a form of reentry, but...well, see NOTE below.

NOTE: The "Maze" surgical procedure cuts (and resutures) the atria into a maze of channels that provides a continuous pathway from the SA Node to the AV Node. This procedure eliminates any possibility of reentry circuits. Yet a study of patients recovering from the maze procedure, revealed that 47% developed Atrial Flutter (or Atrial Fibrillation) postoperatively. This raises considerable doubt that the origin of Atrial Flutter could be reentry.

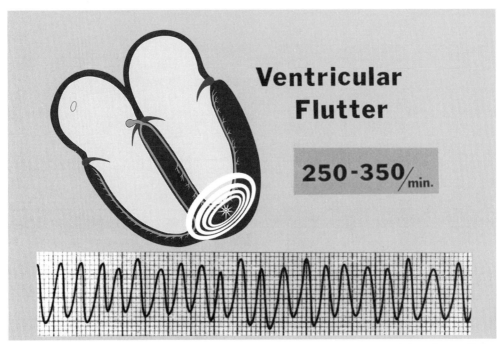

Ventricular Flutter is produced by a single ventricular automaticity focus firing at an exceptionally rapid rate of 250 to 350 per minute. It has a smooth sine-wave appearance with no jagged waves.

Ventricular Flutter is caused by a highly irritable ventricular focus that is desperately discharging at a rate of _____ to _____ per minute.

250
350

The ventricular rate in ventricular flutter is so rapid that the _____ hardly have enough time to fill – even partially, so this arrhythmia rapidly deteriorates into a deadly arrhythmia.

ventricles

The smooth _____-wave pattern of ventricular flutter is its distinguishing characteristic. The appearance is as important as its rate. Ventricular Flutter is nearly always a prelude to a deadly arrhythmia...see next page.

sine

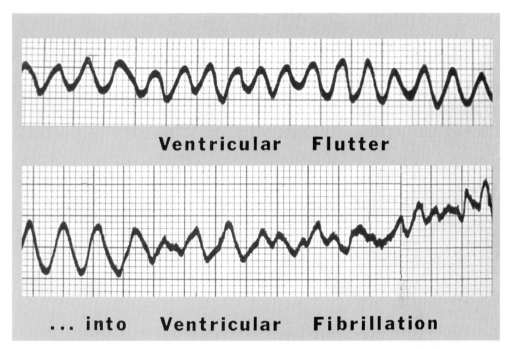

True Ventricular Flutter almost invariably deteriorates into Ventricular Fibrillation which requires immediate Cardio-Pulmonary Resuscitation and defibrillation.

NOTE: During Ventricular Flutter, the ventricles are contracting at an alarming rate. The above (continuous but separated) tracing shows Ventricular Flutter at a rate of about 300 per minute, which is five contractions per second. Blood is a viscous fluid, and the ventricles cannot properly fill (and empty) at a rate of 5 times per second; in fact they hardly fill at all. For this reason there is no effective cardiac output. Therefore, the coronary arteries are not receiving blood, and the heart itself has no blood supply. Ventricular fibrillation results, as many profoundly hypoxic ventricular automaticity foci desperately try in vain to compensate.

PRACTICE TRACING

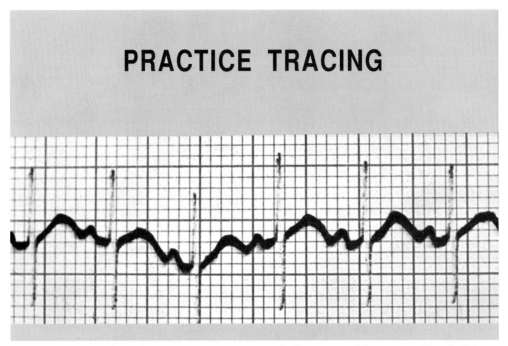

A monitored patient became very concerned about a sudden pounding in his chest.

By the history and the rate (which you determined by observation), you identify the rhythm as a paroxysmal _____ . Now you must determine the causative irritable automaticity focus.   tachycardia

Because this paroxysmal tachycardia has narrow, normal looking QRS's, it could <u>not</u> have originated in an irritable _____ focus; therefore it must be some type of supraventricular tachycardia.   ventricular

There appear to be P' waves present, so we are probably dealing with an automaticity focus in the _____. (You have already ruled out a Junctional focus, because any retrograde depolarizations that it might have produced, would record as inverted P' waves, which are usually adjacent to the QRS when they precede it).   atria

NOTE: This is Paroxysmal Atrial Tachycardia (PAT) and because each P' wave produces a QRS response, it could not be PAT with block. Quickly review the illustrations for the paroxysmal tachycardias before we go on.

Fibrillation

multiple foci rapidly discharge

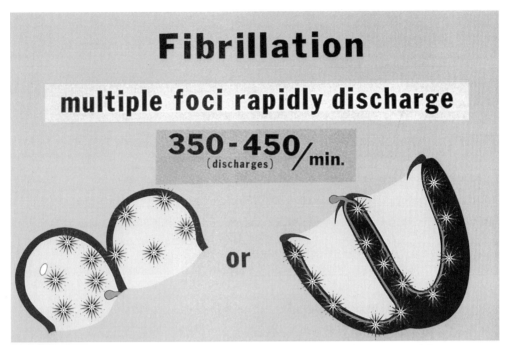

350-450(discharges)/**min.**

or

"Fibrillation" is a totally erratic rhythm caused by continuous, rapid rate discharges from numerous automaticity foci in either the atria or in the ventricles.

NOTE: Fibrillation is caused by rapid discharges from numerous profoundly irritable automaticity foci in the atria (Atrial Fibrillation), or due to numerous profoundly irritable foci in the ventricles rapidly discharging (Ventricular Fibrillation). Both types represent a pathological condition: these (irritable) foci all suffer from entrance block, therefore they are not overdrive-suppressed, so they all discharge rapidly at once. The resulting rhythm is so erratic and uncoordinated that distinct, complete waves are not distinguishable, thus rates are impossible to determine. The involved chambers merely twitch rapidly.

NOTE: The rate 350 to 450 per minute is not a true rate, since many of the foci discharge simultaneously. Both the number and the tachy-rate of individual foci is conjectural. The range of "rate" is more relative and hypothetical than real, because fibrillating chambers do not effectively pump at all.

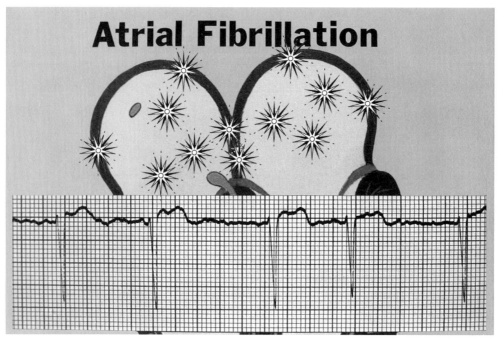

Atrial Fibrillation

Atrial Fibrillation (AF) is caused by many irritable atrial foci (with entrance block) firing at rapid rates producing an exceedingly rapid, erratic atrial rhythm. The atrial "rate" is 350 to 450 per minute. Notice the irregular ventricular response.

Atrial fibrillation occurs when many irritable atrial foci fire rapidly, but since they suffer from entrance block, none of them are overdrive-_____; they all fire rapidly at once to produce   suppressed an excessively rapid series of tiny, erratic spikes on EKG.

NOTE: Only a small portion of the atria is depolarized by any one discharge from an atrial focus, and because so many atrial foci are rapidly firing, no single depolarization spreads very far. Only occasional depolarizations conduct (through the AV Node) to the ventricles, producing a very irregular ventricular rhythm.

NOTE: With a Normal Sinus Rhythm, each pacing impulse that the SA Node generates spreads through the atria like an enlarging, circular wave; much like a pebble dropped into a pool of water. However, the multiple erratic depolarizations of atrial fibrillation are analogous to a rain shower striking the same pool.

Atrial Fibrillation

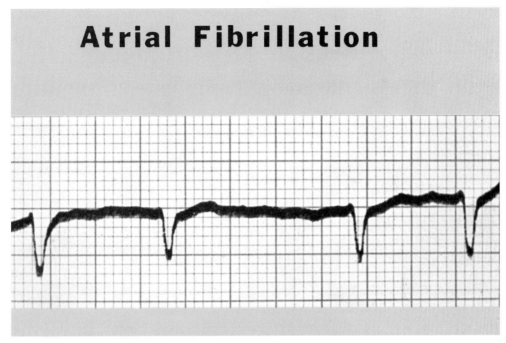

Atrial Fibrillation often appears only as an wavy baseline without P or P' waves. The QRS response is not regular and may be fast or slow.

Atrial Fibrillation may cause such small, erratic spikes that it appears like a wavy baseline without visible __ waves (and without distinguishable P' waves either).   P

The AV Node is irregularly stimulated during atrial fibrillation, so the _____ (QRS) response is irregular. Therefore,   ventricular on EKG the QRS's occur somewhat randomly (the tracing on page 290 also shows this), and the pulse is irregular.

NOTE: The ventricular rate depends on the AV Node's duration of refractoriness after it is stimulated. The AV Node usually allows a relatively normal range of ventricular rate, albeit always *irregular*. Sometimes the AV Node allows an increased number of depolarization stimuli to pass through, producing a rapid ventricular rate that may require pharmacological control.
Always determine the ventricular (pulse) rate (QRS's per 6-second strip times 10) and document it. If the ventricular rate is out of a safe range for the patient, it should be treated appropriately.

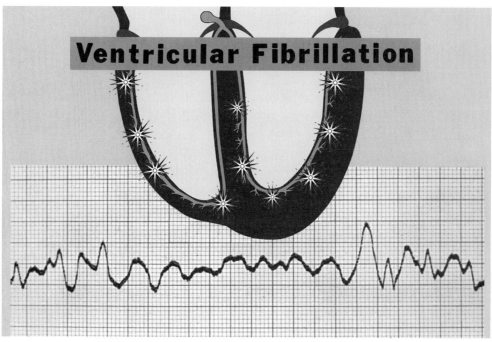

Ventricular Fibrillation (VF) is caused by rapid-rate discharges from many profoundly irritable ventricular automaticity foci, producing an erratic, rapid twitching of the ventricles (ventricular "rate" is 350 to 450 per minute).

Ventricular Fibrillation is due to numerous irritable ventricular foci pacing rapidly (each of them suffering from entrance block, so they can not be _____-suppressed) producing an   overdrive
erratic twitching of the ventricles.

Because there so many ventricular _____ firing rapidly,   foci
each one repeatedly depolarizes only a small area of ventricle.
This results in a rapid, ineffective twitching of the ventricles.

This erratic twitching of VF has been called a "bag of worms," for this is the way the ventricles actually appear. On EKG the tracing is totally erratic, without identifiable _____, and the   waves
ventricles do not provide mechanical pumping.

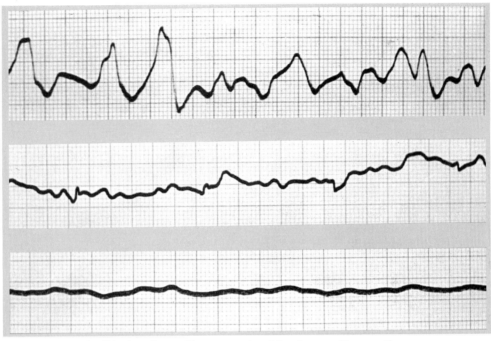

Ventricular Fibrillation is easily recognized by its totally erratic appearance and lack of any identifiable waves on the electrocardiogram.

We recognize Ventricular Fibrillation by its completely erratic appearance on the EKG tracing. Even with large deflections there are no identifiable _____.

waves

There is no predictable pattern of _____ Fibrillation. As you can see, it looks different at every moment, but it is so erratic that it is difficult to miss, thank Goodness.

Ventricular

If you do recognize any repetition of pattern or regularity of deflections, you probably are not dealing with __ __.

VF

NOTE: These three strips are from a continuous tracing of the same patient's dying heart. Notice how the amplitude of the deflections diminishes as the heart dies.

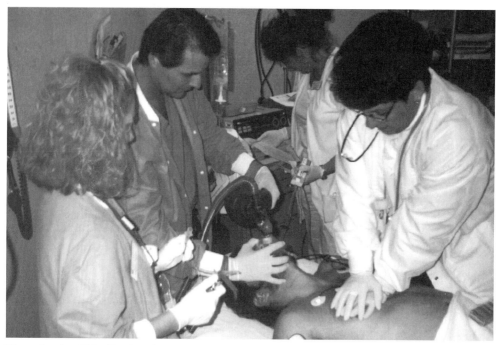

Ventricular Fibrillation is a type of *cardiac arrest,* for there is no pumping action by the heart; this is a dire emergency! VF requires immediate CPR and defibrillation, with a defibrillator or AED (see last paragraph, p. 304).

Ventricular Fibrillation is a type of cardiac _____. There is no   arrest
effective cardiac output, because the ventricles are only twitching
erratically. There is no ventricular pumping, so there is no circulation.

NOTE: There are two other types of cardiac arrest: *Cardiac Standstill* ("Asystole") occurs when there is no detectable cardiac activity on EKG. This is a rare circumstance when the SA Node and the escape mechanisms of all the foci at all levels are unable to assume pacing responsibility. *Pulseless Electrical Activity* (PEA) is present when a dying heart produces weak signs of electrical activity on EKG, but the moribund heart cannot respond mechanically (no detectable pulse).

NOTE: VF requires immediate defibrillation. Cardiac Arrest is an emergency that demands immediate intervention. <u>C</u>ardio-<u>P</u>ulmonary <u>R</u>esuscitation (cardiac massage and assisted respiration) is carried out in order to circulate oxygenated blood by external mechanical means. The technique of CPR was originally taught only to hospital and ambulance personnel, but it is now imperative that every person master this technique. Only when CPR skills are universally known, can all victims of cardiac arrest get immediate lifesaving care at any location. Please review "Fibrillation" illustrations.

164

Heart Blocks

- **Sinus Block**

- **AV Block**

- **Bundle Branch Block**

- **Hemiblock** *(begins page 277)*

Heart Blocks* can occur in the SA Node, the AV Node, or in the larger divisions of the ventricular conduction system.

Heart blocks may develop in any of these areas: the SA _____,   Node
the AV Node, the His Bundle, the Bundle Branches, or in either
of the two subdivisions of the Left Bundle Branch (Hemiblock).

Heart Blocks are blocks of electrical conduction that
prevent (or retard) the passage of _____ stimuli.   depolarization

NOTE: When examining the rhythm on a tracing, ALWAYS
check for all the varieties of Heart Blocks, because the same patient
can have more than one type of block.

* Heart Blocks is a colloquial term, which is more commonly referred to simply as "Blocks"
  in medical circles.

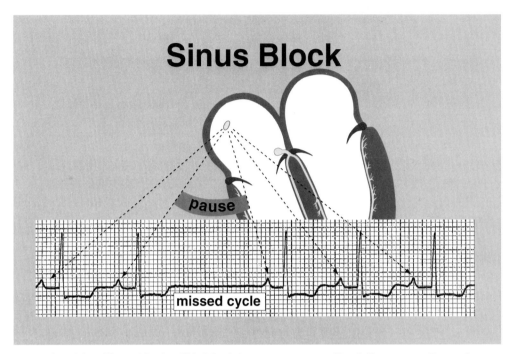

Sinus Block

pause

missed cycle

An unhealthy Sinus Node (SA Node) may temporarily fail to pace for at least one cycle ("Sinus Block"), but then it resumes pacing. Notice that the missed cycle has no P wave; a very important feature.

With Sinus Block (also called "SA Node Block" or simply "SA Block"), an unhealthy SA Node* stops its pacing activity for at least one complete _____, so the block is usually transient. cycle

After the pause of Sinus Block, pacing resumes at the same rate (and timing) as prior to the block, since the SA Node resumes its pacing responsibility in step with its previous rhythm. However, the pause may produce an <u>escape</u> <u>beat</u> from an automaticity _____. focus

NOTE: The P waves before and after the pause are identical because the SA Node continues to generate atrial depolarization with the same timing as before. But a long pause may elicit an escape beat from an automaticity focus before the SA Node can resume pacing.

* Some experts claim that the SA Node does generate a stimulus, but that it is blocked from exiting the SA Node. This is referred to as "Sinus Exit Block".

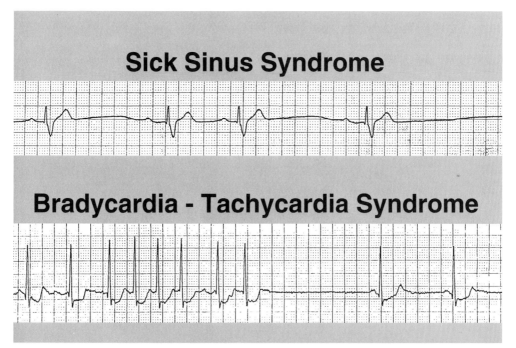

Sick Sinus Syndrome

Bradycardia - Tachycardia Syndrome

Sick Sinus Syndrome (SSS) is a wastebasket of arrhythmias caused by SA Node dysfunction, associated with unresponsive supraventricular (atrial and Junctional) automaticity foci that are also dysfunctional and can't employ their normal escape mechanism.

NOTE: Sick Sinus Syndrome most often occurs in elderly individuals who have heart disease. It is usually characterized by marked Sinus Bradycardia, but without the normal escape mechanisms by atrial and Junctional foci. SSS may also present as recurrent episodes of Sinus Block or Sinus Arrest associated with faulty (or absent) escape mechanisms of all supraventricular foci.

NOTE: Because of the exclusive parasympathetic innervation to the SA Node and all supraventricular (atrial and Junctional) foci, excessive parasympathetic activity depresses the pacing rate of the SA Node, and depresses the atrial and Junctional foci as well. Therefore, young, healthy individuals (e.g., conditioned athletes like marathon runners) who often have parasympathetic hyperactivity at rest, appear to have convincing signs of SSS (*pseudo Sick Sinus Syndrome*).

NOTE: Patients with SSS may develop intermittent episodes of SVT (sometimes even Atrial Flutter or Atrial Fibrillation) mingled with the Sinus Bradycardia. This is *Bradycardia-Tachycardia Syndrome*.

AV BLOCK

1° (first degree) AV Block

2° (second degree) AV Block

3° (third degree) AV Block

Atrio-Ventricular (AV) *Block,* when minimal, delays the impulse (descending from the atria) within the AV Node, making a longer-than-normal pause before ventricular stimulation. More serious AV Blocks may totally block some (or all) atrial stimuli from reaching the ventricles.

In its most innocuous form, an ___ Block delays the atrial impulse   AV
before depolarization is conducted to the ventricular myocardium.

NOTE: You will recall that there is a brief pause between atrial depolarization and ventricular depolarization. This pause between the P wave and the QRS complex lengthens* on the EKG tracing when a minor AV Block is present. More serious AV Blocks completely block some (or all) impulses from reaching the ventricles (on EKG, a P wave with no QRS response).

NOTE: Conventionally recognized varieties of AV Block are:
- *first degree* (1°) *AV Block*
- *second degree* (2°) *AV Block*
- *third degree* (3°) *AV Block*

I will use their alternate designations (in parentheses) so that you will become familiar with both ways of expressing each type of block, since both designations are common in current literature.

*This lengthening is manifested as a prolonged PR interval (see next page).

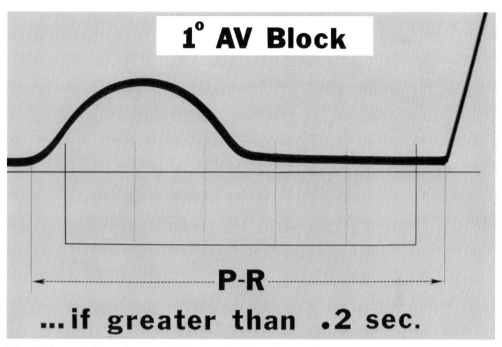

1° AV Block

P-R

...if greater than .2 sec.

The delay of *first degree (1°) AV Block* prolongs the *PR interval* more than one large square (.2 sec.) on EKG.

NOTE: Technically, a "segment" is a portion of baseline, while an "interval" contains at least one wave. So the PR interval includes the P wave and the baseline that follows, up to the point where the QRS complex begins.
The PR interval is measured from the beginning of the P wave to the beginning of the QRS complex.

The delay caused by 1° AV Block prolongs the ___ interval.   PR

The PR interval normally should be less than one large square
which is less than ___ second.   .2
                                                                                            (2/10)

NOTE: You must observe (measure and record) the PR interval on every EKG, for if the PR interval is longer than one large square, some kind of AV Block is present.

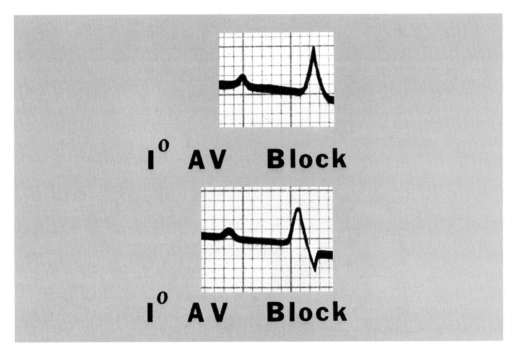

A *first degree AV Block* is characterized by a PR interval greater than .2 sec. (one large square). The amount of PR prolongation is consistent with each cycle.

Once you recognize a prolonged PR _____, you should determine the type of AV Block that is present.   interval

Some type of AV Block is present if any PR interval is longer then ___ second.   .2
(two-tenths)

A first degree AV Block is present when the P-QRS-T sequence is consistently normal, but the PR interval is prolonged the same amount in every _____.   cycle

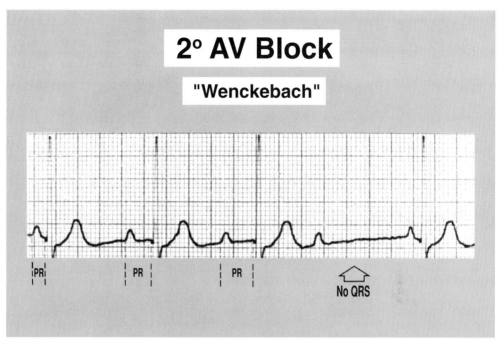

2° AV Block

"Wenckebach"

iPRi | PR | | PR | No QRS

The *Wenckebach phenomenon* is a second degree AV Block in which the PR interval becomes progressively longer from cycle to cycle until the AV Node will no longer conduct a stimulus from above.

The Wenckebach phenomenon (pronounced "Winky-bok") occurs when the AV Block progressively prolongs the PR interval with each successive _____.   cycle

The PR interval becomes gradually longer in successive cycle until the final P wave fails to elicit a ____ response ("dropped QRS").   QRS

The P wave and its associated QRS complex get farther apart in successive cycles. The last __ wave stands alone. Then the pattern   P repeats. This pattern (sometimes called a "Wenckebach footprint") may consist of anywhere from two to eight or more cycles.

NOTE: Wenckebach phenomenon is a type of 2° AV Block that is usually located within the AV Node. Wenckebach is sometimes caused by parasympathetic excess (which slows AV conduction) or drugs that induce or mimic these parasympathetic effects. This is also referred to as *Type I*, 2° AV Block. Because the PR lengthening is gradual from cycle to cycle, you must discipline yourself to scan consecutive cycles routinely for this gradually lengthening PR interval that indicates Wenckebach. Repeating patterns of Wenckebach can produce "group beating" that looks similar to couplets of Premature Beats. (Careful!)

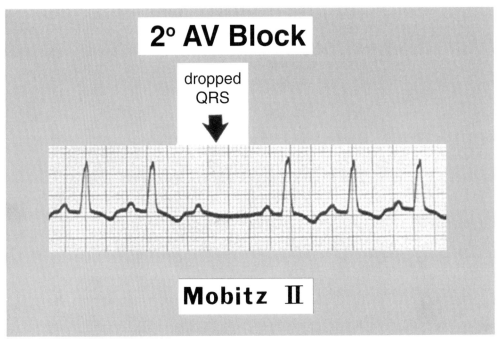

2° AV Block

dropped
QRS

Mobitz II

Occasionally, in an otherwise normal rhythm, a punctual P wave has no QRS response ("dropped QRS"). This is *Mobitz II**, a type of *second degree AV Block*. Usually the other cycles have consistently normal PR intervals.

Mobitz II is noted when a normal, punctual P wave is not followed by a _____ response. The other cycles usually have normal PR intervals.   QRS

NOTE: Mobitz II Block often heralds more serious conduction problems with progressively more involved blocking of ventricular conduction. The Mobitz II block usually develops in the His Bundle or the Bundle Branches.

NOTE: Careful! Do not confuse Mobitz II with a non-conducted PAB or with Sinus Block (in which the entire P-QRS-T cycle is missing). You do not need to memorize patterns (which you might forget), if you understand the basic mechanisms that cause these conspicuous pauses. Just think it through in each case:

- missed P-QRS-T cycle.....SA Node pacing blocked (Sinus Block)
- punctual P wave (no QRS response)....AV conduction is blocked (Mobitz II)
- premature P' wave (no QRS response)....non-conducted PAB

* This is a shortened, colloquial form of the proper nomenclature, "Mobitz, Type II."

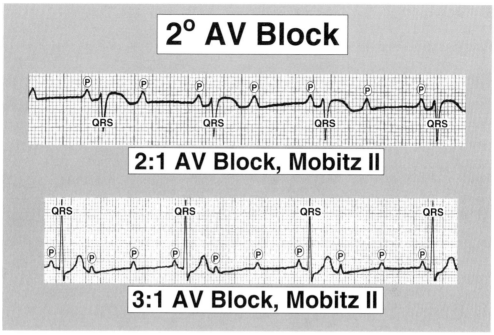

2° AV Block

2:1 AV Block, Mobitz II

3:1 AV Block, Mobitz II

A *Mobitz II* (second degree) AV Block may cause every-other QRS to be blocked causing a 2:1 (two P waves to one QRS) repeating pattern to emerge.

NOTE: Return to the illustration on the previous page and visualize how a repetition of that block pattern becomes the upper tracing on this page (voila!).

A Mobitz II 2° AV Block may appear (at a normal rate) as two P waves to one _____ response, often referred to as "two to one AV Block" (usually written "2:1 AV Block").   QRS

NOTE: Sometimes a Mobitz II (second degree) AV Block requires three atrial depolarizations (P waves) to elicit a single ventricular response (QRS); this is written "3:1 AV Block," which describes the mechanism of conduction. Poorer conduction ratios (e.g., 3:1, 4:1, etc.) relate to *increased severity* of the block, and are sometimes called "advanced Mobitz II AV Block."

WARNING! With Mobitz II, every cycle missing its QRS has a regular, punctual P wave — but NEVER a premature P' wave (see NOTE, page 124). This distinction is critical!!

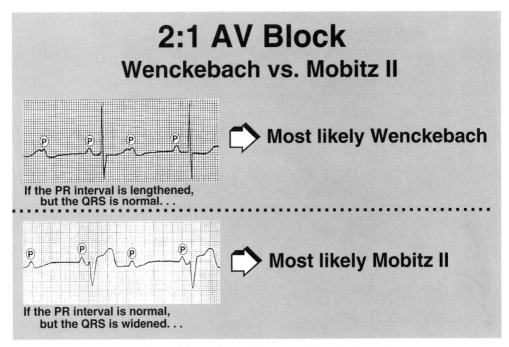

2:1 AV Block
Wenckebach vs. Mobitz II

Most likely Wenckebach

If the PR interval is lengthened,
but the QRS is normal. . .

Most likely Mobitz II

If the PR interval is normal,
but the QRS is widened. . .

Both Wenckebach and Mobitz II have "dropped QRS's", so how can we differentiate between a 2:1 Wenckebach and a 2:1 Mobitz II? We can't always tell the difference, but there are some very telling clues that can be helpful.

NOTE: On EKG a 2:1 AV Block could be considered to be a short, two-cycle Wenckebach pattern. For example, if the first cycle is fairly normal but the PR lengthening in the second cycle is just enough to prevent conduction through the AV Node, this is 2:1 Wenckebach. But by its appearance, you might also interpret the same 2:1 block as a Mobitz II (which is usually the first thing that you think of. Perhaps the following will help...

Because Wenckebach commonly originates in the AV _____,   Node
a 2:1 AV Block of this origin often has an initial lengthened PR
with no wide QRS pattern* (typical of Bundle Branch Block).

And since Mobitz II Block originates below the AV _____, in the   Node
His Bundle or Bundle Branches, we recognize that it often has a
normal PR with a widened QRS (Bundle Branch Block) pattern*.

NOTE: Because Wenckebach is usually innocuous, and Mobitz II is often an early warning sign of impending Complete AV Block (see pages 285-286), differentiating between these two types of 2:1 AV Block is clinically quite important, when we can make the distinction.

* The wide QRS pattern, typical of Bundle Branch Block, is soon explained (pages 177-187).

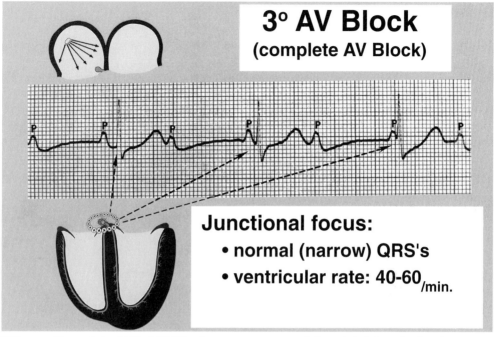

3° AV Block
(complete AV Block)

Junctional focus:
- **normal (narrow) QRS's**
- **ventricular rate: 40-60**/min.

When a Complete (3°) AV Block occurs, none of the atrial depolarizations conduct to the ventricles, so an automaticity focus below the block escapes overdrive suppression to pace the ventricles at its inherent rate.

In 3° (Third Degree) AV Block none of the atrial depolarizations conduct to the ventricles, so this is called a _____ AV Block.   Complete

NOTE: If the Complete AV Block is above the AV Junction (i.e., in the upper AV Node), then a Junctional focus, no longer overdrive-suppressed, escapes to pace the ventricles. However, a Complete AV Block below the AV Junction permits only a ventricular focus to pace the ventricles. Think that through.

We find a specific atrial (P wave) rate and an independent, much slower, ventricular (QRS) _____ in third degree AV Block.   rate
This is *AV Dissociation.*

NOTE: The AV Dissociation tips us off that there is a Complete (3°) AV Block. QRS morphology and the ventricular rate help us identify the focus. If the QRS's appear generally normal (because each pacing stimulus passes down the ventricular conduction system), and if the ventricular rate is 40 to 60 per minute (the inherent rate range of Junctional foci), we can assume that the focus pacing ventricles is in the AV Junction ("idio-Junctional rhythm")*. See illustration.

* Pacing of a Junctional focus may accelerate to become an *accelerated idiojunctional rhythm.*

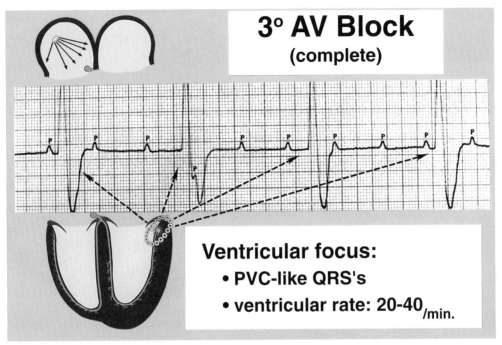

3° AV Block
(complete)

Ventricular focus:
- **PVC-like QRS's**
- **ventricular rate: 20-40**/min.

When a Complete AV Block occurs *below* the AV Junction, a ventricular focus escapes overdrive suppression to pace the ventricles at its slow inherent rate of only 20 to 40 per min.; so slow, in fact, that cerebral blood flow is compromised and syncope may ensue.

Noticing AV Dissociation (separate atrial [P wave] and ventricular [QRS] rates), you must first check the morphology of the QRS's. Here we see large, wide, PVC-like complexes, so we know that the ventricles are probably being paced by a _____ focus.   ventricular

We also see that the ventricular rate is within the inherent rate range (20 to 40 / min.) of a _____ focus.   ventricular

We understand that a ventricular focus could only escape to pace if there were no active AV Junctional _____ to overdrive-suppress it.   focus
So the Complete AV Block must lie below the AV Junction (i.e., below the AV Node). Distinguish this from the previous page.

NOTE: In 3° (Complete) AV Block the ventricular rate may be so slow that blood flow to the brain is inadequate, and the patient may lose consciousness (syncope). This is *Stokes-Adams Syndrome*. Patients with Complete AV Block need continuous surveillance and maintenance of airway ...many die needlessly without. Any patient with Complete AV Block needs an artificial pacemaker.

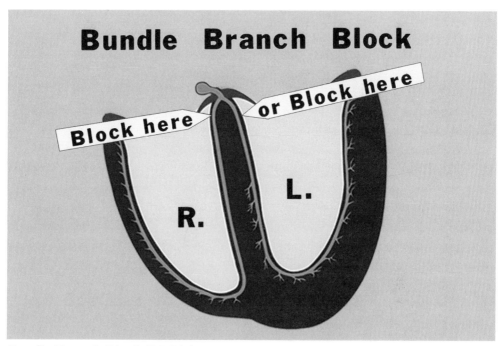

Bundle Branch Block (BBB) is caused by a block (of conduction) in the Right or in the Left Bundle Branch. The blocked Bundle Branch delays depolarization to the ventricle that it supplies.

Normally, the Right Bundle Branch quickly conducts the
stimulus of depolarization to the right ventricle, and the
Left Bundle Branch does the same to the _____ ventricle.   left
The depolarization stimulus is conducted to both ventricles
at the same time (i.e., simultaneously).

A block of one of the Bundle Branches produces a _____   delay
of depolarization in the ventricle which it supplies.

NOTE: Ordinarily both ventricles are depolarized simultaneously. But
with Bundle Branch Block, the unblocked Bundle Branch conducts normally,
while depolarization in the blocked Bundle Branch has to creep slowly through
the surrounding muscle (which conducts more slowly than the specialized
Bundle Branch) to stimulate the Bundle Branch below the block. Below the
block, delayed depolarization proceeds rapidly again. However, the delay in the
blocked Bundle Branch allows the unblocked ventricle to begin depolarizing
before the blocked ventricle.

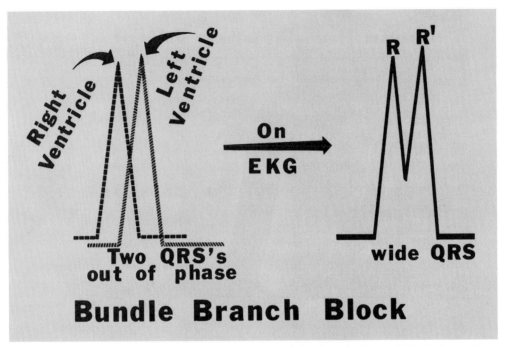

Bundle Branch Block

Therefore in Bundle Branch Block, one ventricle depolarizes slightly later than the other, causing two "joined QRS's" to appear on EKG.

When a Bundle Branch Block is present, either the left or the right ventricle may depolarize late, depending on which Bundle _____ is blocked.   Branch

NOTE: Individual depolarization of the right ventricle and depolarization of the left ventricle are still of normal duration. Because the ventricles do not depolarize simultaneously, this produces the "widened QRS" appearance that we see on the EKG. The two "out-of-sync" QRS's are superimposed on one-another, and the machine records this combined electrical activity as a widened QRS.

NOTE: Because the "widened QRS" represents the non-simultaneous depolarization of both ventricles (one punctually depolarized, the other slightly delayed), we usually see two R waves named in sequential order: R and R'. The R' (pronounced "R-prime") represents delayed depolarization of the blocked ventricle.

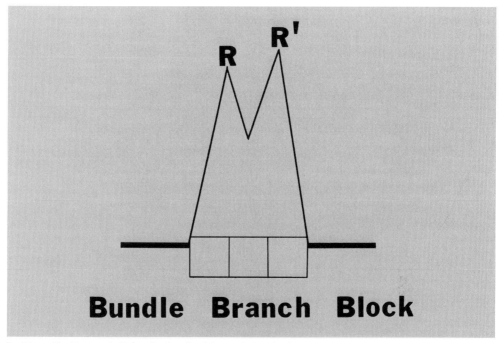

Bundle Branch Block

In Bundle Branch Block the "widened QRS" increases in duration to three small squares (.12 sec.) or greater, and two R waves (R and R') appear. The R' designates the delayed depolarization of the blocked side.

NOTE: Simultaneous depolarization of the ventricles normally occurs in less than twelve hundredths second, producing a QRS that is less than three small squares in duration.

The diagnosis of Bundle Branch Block is mainly based on the widened _____ (.12 sec. or more duration).   QRS

In order to make the diagnosis of Bundle Branch Block, the QRS complex should be at least _____ small squares wide (.12 sec.).   three (3) Check the QRS width of every EKG that you read!

NOTE: The needle that records the EKG tracing moves rapidly enough to record most of the heart's electrical activity accurately. However, with great deflections the needle lags a bit mechanically, sometimes giving us an exaggerated duration on the tracing. Therefore, it is best to check the limb leads for QRS duration (where deflections are minimal) rather than the chest leads where the QRS deflections are great.

NOTE: If a patient with BBB develops a supraventricular tachycardia, the rapid succession of widened QRS's may imitate Ventricular Tachycardia. Careful!

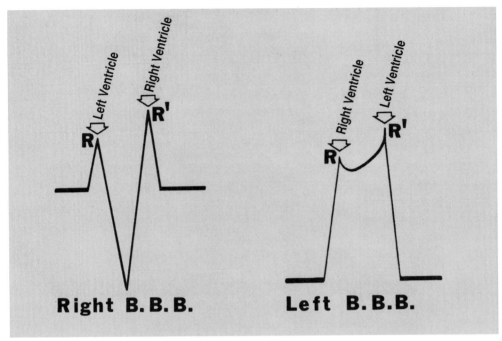

Right B.B.B.   **Left B.B.B.**

In *Left Bundle Branch Block* (LBBB), left ventricular depolarization is delayed. In *Right Bundle Branch Block* (RBBB), right ventricular depolarization is delayed.

In Bundle Branch Block you first notice the widened _____ complex. Then you should be able to find the R,R' configuration in the chest leads.

QRS

In Right Bundle Branch Block the left ventricle depolarizes punctually, so the R represents left ventricular depolarization, and the R' represents delayed _____ ventricular depolarization.

right

In Left Bundle Branch Block, left ventricular depolarization is delayed, so the right ventricle depolarizes punctually (R), and the R' represents delayed _____ ventricular depolarization.

left

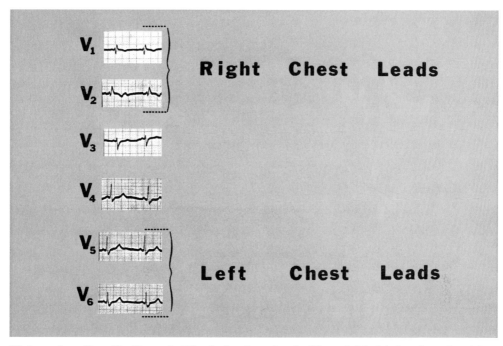

If there is a Bundle Branch Block, look at leads V_1 and V_2 (right chest leads) and leads V_5 and V_6 (left chest leads) for the R,R'.

When the QRS complex is wide enough to make the diagnosis of BBB, we immediately look at the right and left chest leads for the ____.   R,R'

NOTE: During ventricular depolarization and just afterward (up to the peak of the T wave), any additional stimulus cannot depolarize the ventricles, that is, they are *refractory* to a premature stimulus. The Bundle Branches have a refractory period, but occasionally their refractory periods are not identical, so with a supraventricular tachycardia one Bundle Branch is receptive to stimulation before the other. At a certain *critical* rapid rate one Bundle Branch conducts before the other, so this *rate-dependent* Bundle Branch Block produces a tachycardia with wide QRS's that imitates Ventricular Tachycardia.

The right chest leads are V_1 and ___. V_2

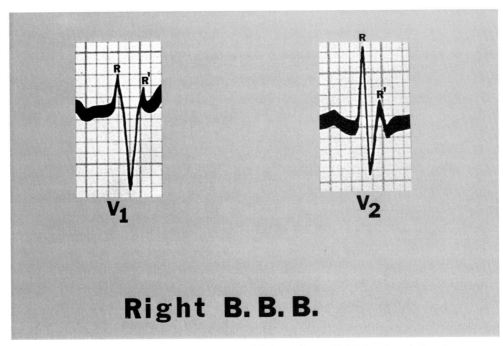

Right B. B. B.

There is a Right Bundle Branch Block if there is an R,R' in the right chest leads, V$_1$ or V$_2$.

With a wide _____ (and a diagnosis of BBB), check the right and left chest leads for R,R'.

QRS

Then, if there is an R,R' in the right chest leads V$_1$ or V$_2$ this is probably a _____ Bundle Branch Block.

Right

In Right Bundle Branch Block, the right ventricle is depolarizing slightly later than the left ventricle, so the R' in the above illustration represents the delayed depolarization to the (blocked) _____ ventricle.

right

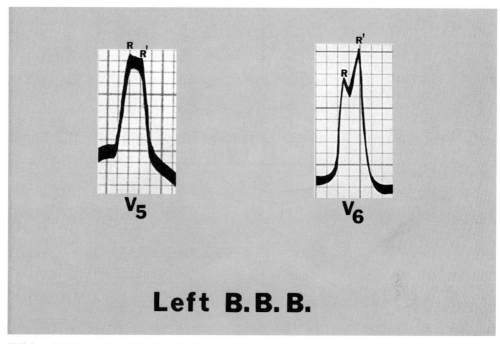

Left B.B.B.

With a BBB an R,R' in the left chest leads V_5 or V_6 means that Left Bundle Branch Block is present, and the R' represents delayed depolarization of the *left* ventricle.

The chest electrode is located over the left ventricle in
left chest leads _____ and V_6. V_5

Occasionally, the R,R' in V_5 or V_6 will appear only as a
flattened peak with two tiny points in _____ Bundle   Left
Branch Block. (Examine the QRS in V_5 in the illustration).

In LBBB the right ventricle depolarizes before the left ventricle,
so the first portion of the wide QRS represents _____   right
ventricular depolarization.

NOTE: Compare and make a mental note of the typical pattern (i.e., shape) of Right and Left BBB. These patterns are important because sometimes a PVC or the ventricular complexes in VT are said to have a RBBB or LBBB pattern, and you should understand what that means.

NOTE: The Left Bundle Branch has two subdivisions ("fascicles") and blocks of these fascicles are called *Hemiblocks* (pages 278 - 286).

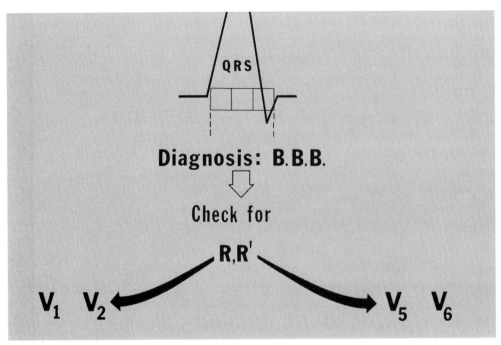

Remember, if there is a wide QRS (three small squares), you should identify
which Bundle Branch is blocked by checking the left and right chest leads.

To diagnose BBB the QRS complex must be at least ___ of a   .12
second in duration. Just for smiles, let's identify the type of BBB
in the illustration on page 181.

NOTE: In some individuals recovery from refractoriness (during the last stage
of repolarization) differs slightly in duration between bundle branches. So only
at a particular critical rate of tachycardia, one ventricle depolarizes after the
other to produce a *rate-dependent* Bundle Branch Block (see NOTE, page 181).

The R,R' pattern may occur in only one chest _____. It is   lead
often difficult to see the R', but usually it can be found in the
right chest leads V_1 or V_2 or in the left chest leads V_5 or V_6.

NOTE: Occasionally you will see an R,R' in a QRS of normal duration. This
is called "incomplete" BBB.

184

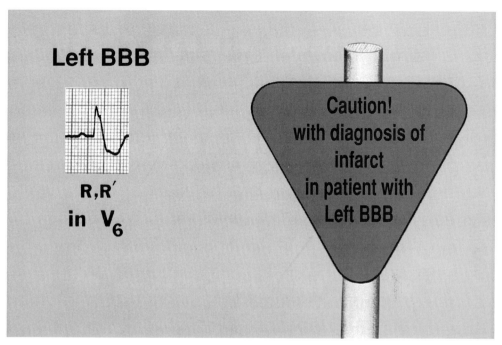

Left BBB

R,R′
in V$_6$

Caution!
with diagnosis of
infarct
in patient with
Left BBB

IMPORTANT: With *Left Bundle Branch Block* one cannot accurately diagnose infarction on EKG.

NOTE: With Left Bundle Branch Block the left ventricle depolarizes late, so the first portion of the QRS complex represents right ventricular electrical activity. Therefore we cannot identify significant Q waves (which identify infarction) originating in the left ventricle, for they would be buried in the middle of the QRS.

However, the EKG should be examined for signs of infarction in the presence of _____ Bundle Branch Block, which has no effect on the diagnosis.   Right

NOTE: With Left Bundle Branch Block other studies are needed to verify the presence of acute myocardial infarction.

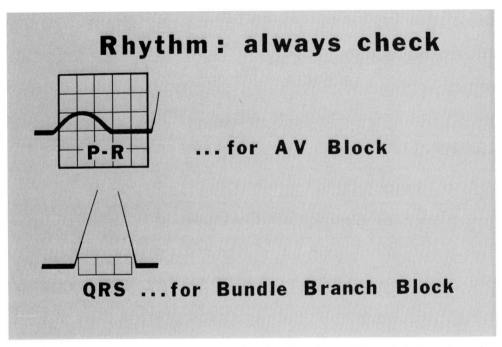

Rhythm: always check

P-R   ...for **AV Block**

QRS ...for Bundle Branch Block

Remember that you must always check* the duration of the PR intervals and the duration of the QRS complex when examining the rhythm on an EKG.

You must always check* the PR intervals on all EKG's, because if <u>any</u> is prolonged more than one large square, then there is some kind of ___ Block present (and, of course, look for missing QRS's,   AV which indicate that a 2° or 3° AV Block is present).

The QRS duration must be checked* on all EKG's, for if it is prolonged to .12 second or _____ there is a Bundle Branch Block.   more

NOTE: Always check the PR intervals and the QRS duration when scrutinizing the rhythm on any EKG. This must be part of any EKG interpretation. The spontaneous appearance of Mobitz II AV Block or Bundle Branch Block may be an early warning of impending infarction.

NOTE: *Hemiblocks* usually result from infarction, so they are described in the Infarction chapter. A hemiblock is a block of one of the two divisions ("fascicles") of the Left Bundle Branch.

*Once you "check" these criteria on EKG, you should record the precise PR and QRS duration.

Bundle Branch Block

Vector : ?

Ventricular Hypertrophy?

The Mean QRS Vector (Axis) and ventricular hypertrophy cannot be determined accurately in the presence of Bundle Branch Block.

NOTE: Because the Mean QRS Vector represents the general direction of the simultaneous depolarization of the ventricles, it is very difficult to represent such a vector in BBB. This is because the ventricles are depolarizing in sequence, and there are really two separate (right and left) ventricular vectors.

NOTE: The criteria for ventricular hypertrophy (enlargement) are based on a normal QRS. Bundle Branch Block produces large QRS deflections because each ventricle lacks the (usual) simultaneous electrical opposition from depolarization of the other ventricle. Therefore the diagnosis of ventricular hypertrophy should be very guarded with BBB. However, atrial hypertrophy can be diagnosed in the presence of BBB.

PRACTICE TRACING

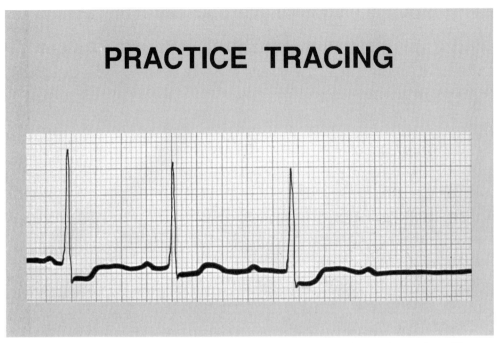

An examining physician noticed that his patient had an irregular pulse. He was surprised to feel a group of three pulse beats followed by a pause, and this group of beats seemed to repeat over and over. Let's share the EKG.

On the EKG we notice that the last full cycle in each group has a PR interval that exceeds .2 sec., so we suspect some kind of ___ Block.

AV

After the last full cycle we notice a lone P wave with no _____ response.

QRS

Upon close examination we note that the PR interval is normal at first, but becomes progressively longer with each successive cycle. We now recognize _____ phenomenon, which is a type of 2° AV Block.

Wenckebach

NOTE: Now is the time to review the illustrations on pages 165 to 188.

NOTE: Review rhythm by turning to the **Personal Quick Reference Sheets** at the end of this book (pages 312 to 315) and establish your methodology for reading EKG's (page 310).

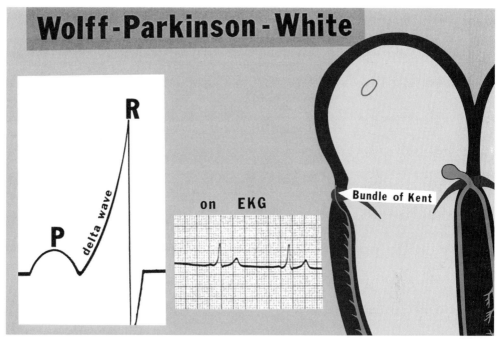

Wolff-Parkinson-White

on EKG

Bundle of Kent

An abnormal, accessory AV conduction pathway can "short circuit" the (usual) delay of ventricular conduction in the AV Node. This prematurely depolarizes ("pre-excites") a portion of the ventricles (producing a delta wave on EKG) just before normal ventricular depolarization is initiated.

The accessory Bundle of _____ causes ventricular   Kent
pre-excitation in *Wolff-Parkinson-White* (WPW) syndrome.

The delta wave creates the illusion of a "shortened" PR interval
and "lengthened" QRS. The delta wave actually records the
depolarization of an area of _____ pre-excitation.   ventricular

NOTE: WPW syndrome is very important because persons
with such an accessory pathway can have paroxysmal tachycardia
by three possible mechanisms:
- re-entry — ventricular depolarization may immediately restimulate the atria
  in a retrograde fashion via the accessory pathway causing a theoretical
  circus re-entry loop.
- rapid conduction — supraventricular tachycardia (including atrial flutter or
  atrial fibrillation) may be rapidly conducted 1:1 through this accessory
  pathway producing dangerously high ventricular rates.
- some Kent Bundles have been found to contain automaticity foci that can
  initiate a paroxysmal tachycardia.

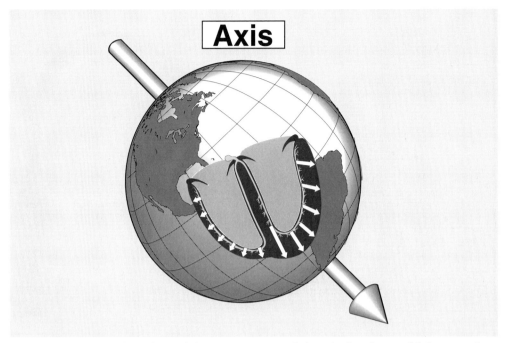

Axis refers to the direction of the movement of depolarization, which spreads throughout the heart to stimulate the myocardium to contract.

NOTE: The axis around which the earth rotates has nothing to do with electrocardiography, but we can borrow the large arrow ("Axis") in the illustration.

The progressive depolarization of the _____ moves in a certain direction.   myocardium

Axis refers to the _____ of depolarization as it passes through the heart.   direction

Direction Of
Vector
Electrical Stimulus

To demonstrate the direction in which depolarization is moving, we use an arrow that is called a "vector".

We can demonstrate the general direction of the movement
of depolarization by using a _____.   vector

The vector shows the direction in which
_____ is moving.   depolarization

When interpreting EKG's, a vector shows the
general _____ of depolarization in the heart.   direction

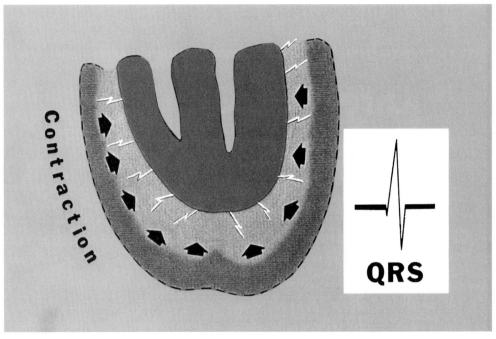

The QRS complex represents the depolarization of the ventricular myocardium.

The QRS complex represents the simultaneous
depolarization of both _____.   ventricles

Ventricular depolarization and contraction can be said
to occur at the same time (but we know that _____   contraction
lasts a little longer).

Depolarization of the ventricles and their contraction
is represented by the _____ complex.   QRS

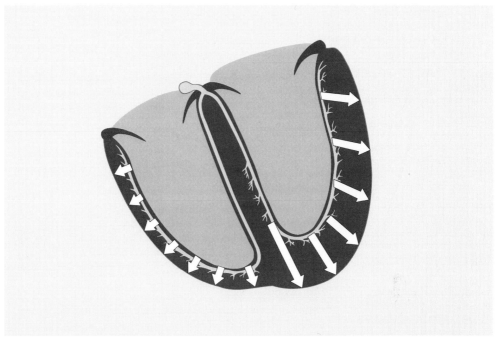

We can use small vectors to demonstrate ventricular depolarization, which begins at the endocardium that lines both ventricles and proceeds toward the outside surface (epicardium) in all areas at once.

NOTE: Once depolarization is beyond the AV Node, the ventricular conduction system conducts this stimulus to the ventricles with great speed. In this way ventricular depolarization begins at the endocardial lining of the ventricles and proceeds through the thickness of the ventricular wall in all areas at about the same time. (We will not yet address depolarization of the ventricular septum).

The Purkinje fibers transmit depolarization to the myocardial cells just beneath the endocardium that lines both ventricles; this occurs so fast, that depolarization begins at the general level of the _____ in all areas at about the same time.   endocardium

Depolarization of the ventricles generally proceeds from the endocardial lining to the outside (epicardial) surface through the full thickness of the_____ wall in all areas at once.   ventricular
(See small vectors in the illustration).

   NOTE: Notice that the thicker left ventricular wall has larger vectors.

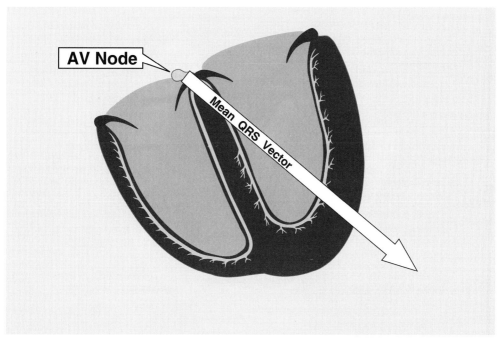

If we add up all the small vectors of ventricular depolarization (*considering both direction and magnitude*), we have one large "Mean QRS Vector" which represents the general direction of ventricular depolarization.

The Mean QRS Vector is the sum of all the smaller vectors of _____ depolarization.

ventricular

By convention we consider the origin of the Mean QRS Vector to be the AV Node, so the "tail" of the Vector is always the ___ _____.

AV Node

Because the small depolarization vectors of the thicker left ventricle are larger (previous page), the Mean QRS Vector points more toward the _____.

left

NOTE: Remember that a vector represents both direction and magnitude of depolarization...bigger vectors represent greater magnitude.

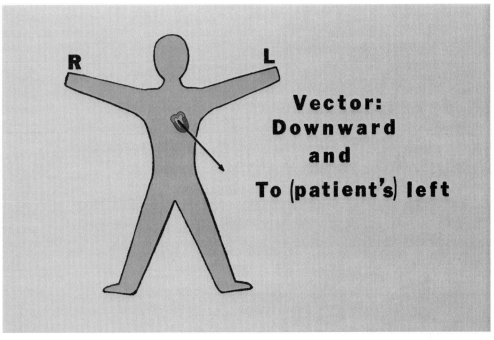

The Mean QRS Vector normally points downward and to the patient's left, because this is the general direction of ventricular depolarization.

The ventricles are in the left side of the chest and angle downward and to the _____.

left

The _____ ____ Vector points downward and toward the patient's left side.

Mean QRS

NOTE: From now on, we occasionally will use the word "Vector" (with a capital "V") to represent the Mean QRS Vector, which depicts the general direction and magnitude of ventricular depolarization. Visualize the Vector over the patient's chest, and remember that it begins in the AV Node.

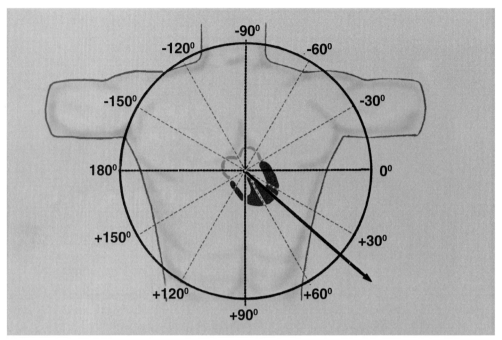

The position of the Mean QRS Vector is described in degrees within a circle drawn over the patient's chest. This circle is in the *frontal* plane. The limb leads are used to determine the position ("Axis") of the Mean QRS Vector in the frontal plane.

We can locate the position of the Mean QRS Vector
within a large _____ around the heart.   circle

The center of the circle is the ____ _____ .   AV Node

The Vector normally points downward and to the patient's
left, that is, between 0 and ____ degrees.   +90
                                                                  (don't forget the +)

NOTE: The "axis" of the heart is simply the Mean QRS Vector when located by degrees in the frontal plane. For example, the axis of the heart in the above illustration is about +40 degrees. Review the illustration and note that 0° is on the patient's left, and that the lower half of the circle is "positive" degrees. The top half of the circle is "negative" degrees.

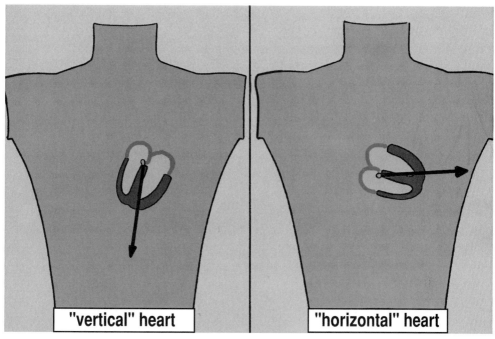

| "vertical" heart | "horizontal" heart |

If the heart is displaced, the Mean QRS Vector is also displaced in the same direction. The AV Node is always the tail of the Vector.

If the heart is rotated toward the patient's _____ side, then the Mean QRS Vector moves toward the right as well. (See illustration).

right

In very obese people the diaphragm is pushed up (and also the heart), so the Mean QRS Vector may point directly to the patient's _____. (See illustration).

left

The tail of the Vector is the ____ _____ .

AV Node

NOTE: In obese individuals the increased abdominal pressure often pushes the diaphragm upward so the position of the displaced heart may be called a "horizontal heart". By the same token, a tall, slender individual may have a so called "vertical heart".

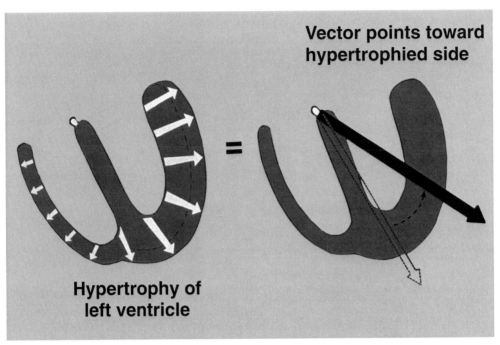

Vector points toward hypertrophied side

Hypertrophy of left ventricle

With hypertrophy (enlargement) of one ventricle, the greater depolarization activity of the hypertrophied side displaces the Mean QRS Vector toward the hypertrophied side.

There is increased depolarization in a _____   hypertrophied
ventricle.

So the Mean QRS Vector deviates toward the _____   ventricle
that is hypertrophied.

NOTE: A hypertrophied ventricle has more (and larger)
vectors, which draw the Mean QRS Vector in that direction.

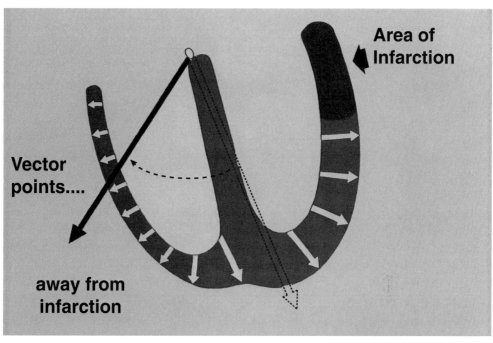

In myocardial infarction there is a necrotic (dead) area of the heart that has lost its blood supply and does not depolarize. The unopposed vectors from the other side draw the Mean QRS Vector away from the infarct.

NOTE: Myocardial infarction occurs when a branch of one of the coronary arteries (the heart's own source of blood supply) becomes occluded. The area of myocardium supplied by this blocked coronary artery has no blood supply and becomes electrically dead (can't depolarize).

In myocardial infarction (coronary occlusion) there is an area in the ventricles that has no _____ supply. This   blood infarcted area cannot depolarize, and therefore it has no vectors.

Since there is no depolarization (and no vectors) in the infarcted area, the vectors from the opposite side are unopposed, so the Mean QRS Vector tends to point away from the _____.   infarct

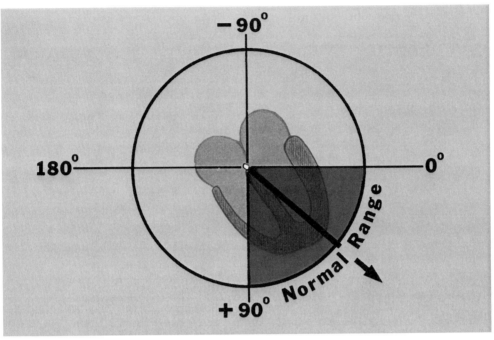

Now you understand why the Mean QRS Vector is diagnostically so valuable. "Axis" is the Mean QRS Vector when given in degrees, and the normal axis range is 0 to +90° in the frontal plane.

The Mean QRS Vector should point downward and to
the patient's _____, that is, in the 0 to +90° range.   left
This is the range of normal axis.

The Mean QRS Vector gives us valuable information
about the position of the _____, and...   heart

...insight into ventricular _____, and   hypertrophy
it also provides us with valuable information concerning
myocardial _____.   infarction

NOTE: The Mean QRS Vector tends to point <u>toward</u> <u>ventricular</u> <u>hypertrophy</u>, and <u>away</u> <u>from</u> <u>myocardial</u> <u>infarction</u>. These basic principles of axis are so logical and easy to understand that you should employ this diagnostic* tool whenever a twelve lead EKG is available.

* The diagnosis of Hemiblocks (pages 277-286) is based on changes in QRS Axis.

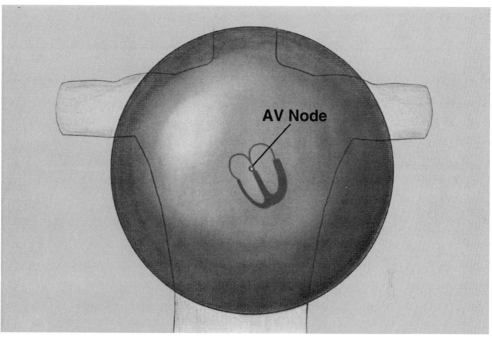

To determine the direction of the Vector, visualize a sphere surrounding the heart, with the AV Node at the center of the sphere.

Visualize a large _____ surrounding the heart.   sphere

The AV Node is the _____ of the sphere.   center

NOTE: The Mean QRS Vector has the AV Node as its tail, and the tip of the arrow touches somewhere on the surface of this hypothetical sphere.

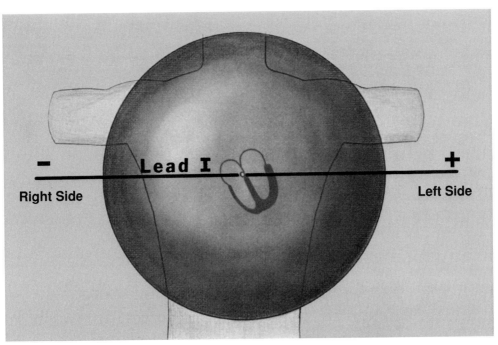

With the sphere in mind, consider lead I (left arm with the positive electrode, right arm with the negative electrode).

Lead I uses the right and left _____ for recording.   arms

If lead I is introduced into the sphere, the patient's left side
(left arm) is _____.   positive

In lead I the right arm is _____.   negative

NOTE: Lead I passes through the center of the sphere, which is the AV Node.

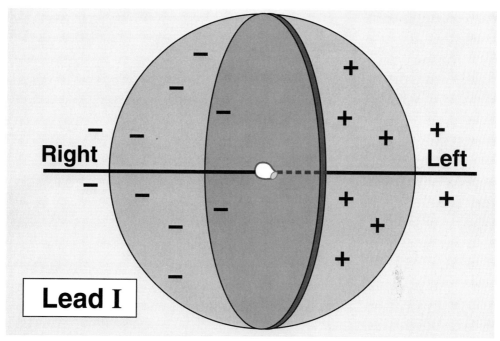

Still considering lead I, the patient's left-hand side of the sphere is positive, and the right half is negative. The center of the sphere is the AV Node.

We are considering only lead ___ at this time.   I

We will now consider the lead I sphere in two _____.   halves

The patient's right half of the sphere is _____.   negative

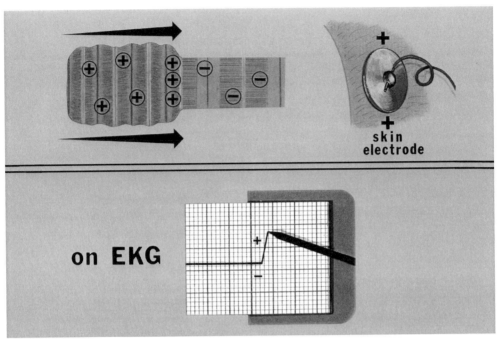

As the positive wave of depolarization within the myocardial cells moves toward a positive (skin) electrode, there is a simultaneous upward (positive) deflection recorded on EKG.

An advancing wave of depolarization may be considered a moving wave of _____ charges.

positive

When this wave of positive charges is moving toward a _____ skin electrode, there is a simultaneous upward (positive) deflection recorded on the EKG.

positive

If you see a _____ (upward) wave on EKG, it means at that instant a depolarization stimulus is moving toward a positive skin electrode that is being used to record the EKG.

positive

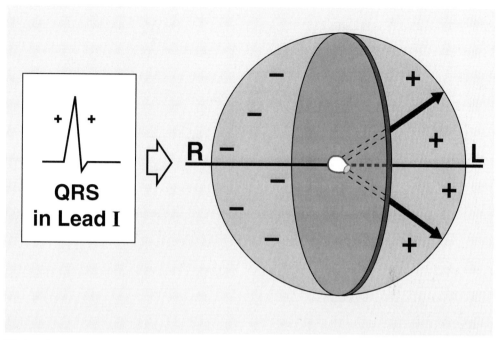

If the QRS complex is POSITIVE (mainly upright) in lead I, the Mean QRS Vector is pointing somewhere into the patient's *left* half (i.e. the positive half) of the sphere.

Obtain an EKG tracing and check the _____ complex in lead I.   QRS

   NOTE: We check the QRS complex because it represents ventricular depolarization on the EKG tracing.

If the QRS in lead I is mainly upright,
it is _____ (positive or negative)...   positive

...and if the QRS is positive in lead I, then the Mean QRS Vector points positively, that is, into the _____ half of the sphere   left
(toward the positive skin electrode on the patient's left arm).

   NOTE: This point becomes clearer if you go back and reread the previous page and continue directly with this page. It comes into focus better on the second go 'round.

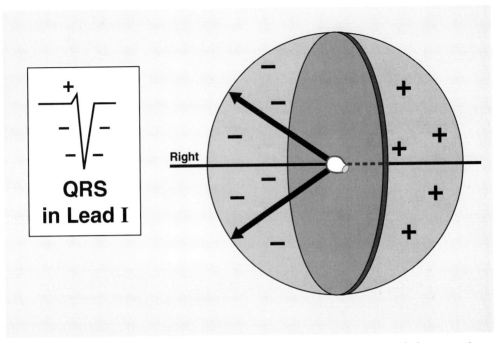

Still considering lead I on the tracing, if the QRS complex is mainly *negative* (downward), the Vector points to the patient's *right* side.

In lead I, if the QRS complex is mainly below the baseline,
it is _____ (positive or negative).   negative

Now checking the lead I sphere surrounding the patient,
a Vector pointing into the negative half of the sphere points
to the patient's _____ side.   right

So if the QRS in lead I is mainly negative, then the Mean
_____ Vector points to the patient's right side (away from   QRS
the positive electrode on the patient's left arm).

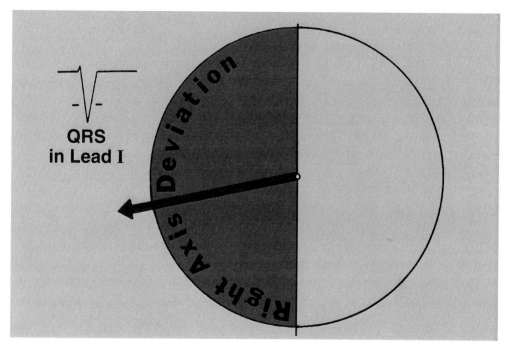

If the QRS is negative in lead I (Vector toward the right), this is *Right Axis Deviation.*

If the Mean QRS Vector points toward the right, we expect the QRS complex in lead I to be _____.

negative

If the Mean QRS Vector points to the patient's right side (to the right of a vertical line drawn through the A V Node), this indicates Right _____ Deviation.

Axis

So if the QRS complex is negative in lead ___, this indicates that there is Right Axis Deviation (R.A.D.).

I

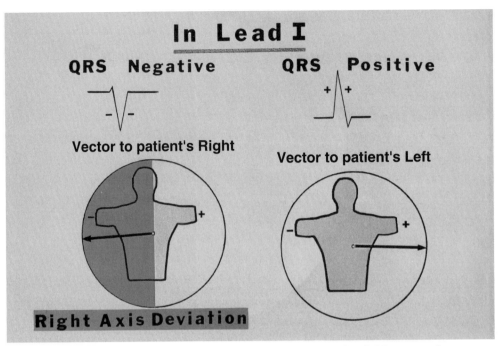

By simple observation, we can tell whether the Mean QRS Vector points to the patient's left or right side.

Lead I is the best lead for detecting Right _____ Deviation.

Axis

If the QRS complex is positive in lead I (which it usually is), this indicates that there is no R.A.D., because the Vector is pointing to the _____ side of the patient.

left

When we record lead I on an EKG, the patient's left arm has the _____ electrode.

positive

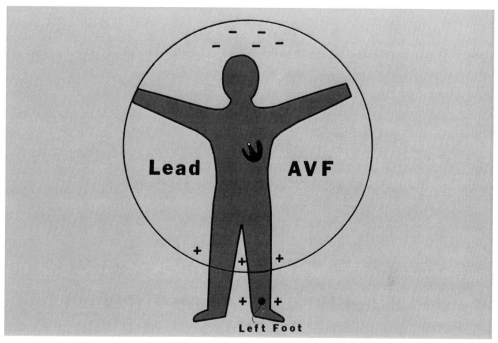

The left foot has a positive electrode in Lead AVF. Imagine a sphere around the patient for lead AVF.

Ignore the lead discussed on the previous page. We are considering only lead _____ at this time.

AVF

NOTE: We are now considering a completely different sphere – the one that surrounds the body when we record lead AVF on the EKG machine. We need to re-orient ourselves as to the positive and negative halves of the sphere in AVF.

When we switch the EKG machine to monitor lead AVF, the machine makes the electrode on the left _____ positive.

foot

The lower half of this sphere is _____.

positive

The center of this sphere is the ___ _____.

AV Node

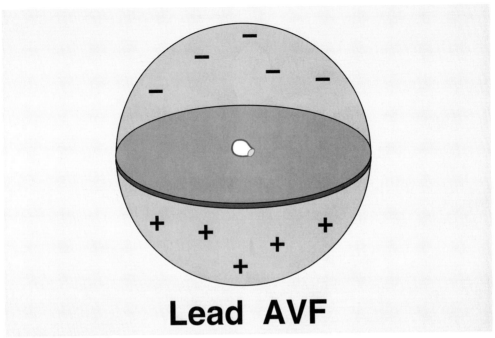

Lead AVF

For AVF the lower half of the sphere is positive, and the upper half is negative.

The lower half of the AVF sphere is the location of the positive
left foot electrode, so we know that the lower half of this sphere is
_____.

positive

The upper portion of the sphere (above the AV Node) is
_____ (positive or negative).

negative

The sphere in AVF has two halves, the upper half is
_____...

negative

...and the lower half of the AVF sphere is _____.

positive

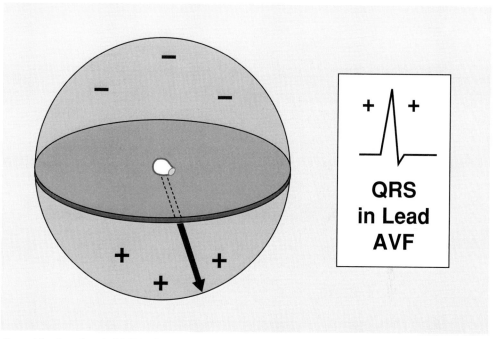

Considering lead AVF of the EKG, if the QRS is mainly positive on the tracing, then the Mean QRS Vector points downward into the positive half of the sphere, toward the positive (lead AVF) electrode.

If the Mean QRS Vector points downward, then the
QRS complex in lead AVF is _____.   upright (or positive)

NOTE: Don't get confused just because the positive QRS is upright,
yet the Vector points downward. You must remember that the Vector
points into the positive half of the sphere when the QRS is positive.
The lower half of the sphere just happens to be the positive half in lead AVF.

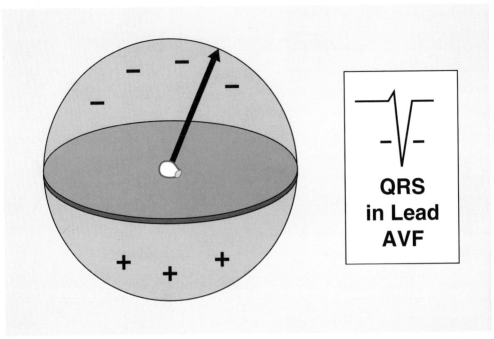

In AVF, if the QRS is negative, the Vector points into the negative half of the sphere.

The center of the sphere is the ___ _____.

AV Node

The upper half of the (lead AVF) sphere is _____.

negative

A negative QRS complex in lead AVF tells us that the Mean QRS Vector points _____ into the negative half of the sphere (i.e., it is pointing away from the positive electrode on the left foot).

upward

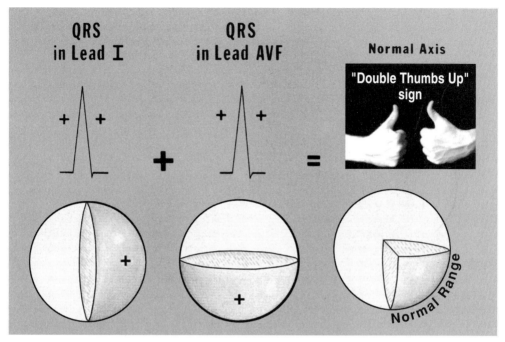

Follow the illustration closely. If the QRS is positive in lead I and also positive in AVF, the Vector points downward and to the patient's left. This is the normal axis range.

A mainly positive QRS in lead I indicates that the Mean
QRS Vector points to the _____ side of the patient and...   left

...a mainly positive QRS complex in lead AVF means
that the Vector points _____.   downward

In the same patient, if the Vector points leftward and also
points downward, the Vector must be in the only quadrant
of the _____ that satisfies both criteria (and it happens   sphere
to be the normal range).

NOTE: Since the ventricles angle downward to the left, and ventricular depolarization moves downward and leftward, it should not surprise you that this is the normal range of the Vector. Remember, Vector position is stated in terms of the patient's left or right. If the QRS is upright in both lead I and AVF (the "double thumbs up sign"), the Vector ("Axis") is within the normal range.

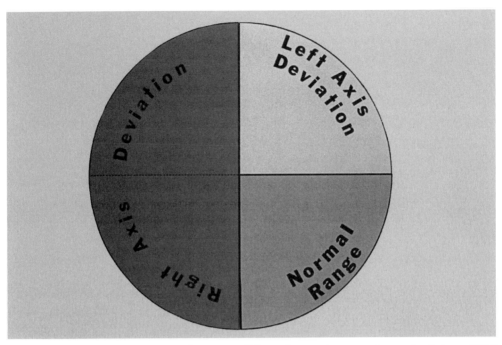

In the frontal plane there are four possible axis quadrants where the Mean QRS Vector may point. Visualize this large circle on the patient's chest in the frontal plane.

NOTE: In the *frontal* plane, we determine if there is any *Deviation* of Axis out of the normal range.

If the Vector points upward (from the AV Node) and to the patient's left, this is Left _____ Deviation (L.A.D.).   Axis

If the Vector points to the patient's right side, this is _____ Axis Deviation (R.A.D.).   Right

If the Vector points downward to the patient's left, it is in the _____ range (i.e., Normal Axis).   normal

NOTE: Remember, Axis is merely the position (that is, the direction) of the Mean QRS Vector, which indicates the general direction of ventricular depolarization.

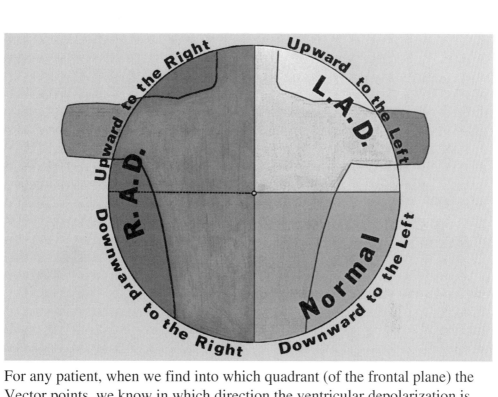

For any patient, when we find into which quadrant (of the frontal plane) the Vector points, we know in which direction the ventricular depolarization is going. The small type in the illustration relates to the patient's right or left.

NOTE: This is how you should visualize the four axis quadrants in a large circle (AV Node is the center) drawn on the patient's chest in the frontal plane. On some EKG charts the Mean QRS Vector is depicted in a similar circle (which represents the frontal plane).

The upper left quadrant represents _____ Axis Deviation (L.A.D.).

Left

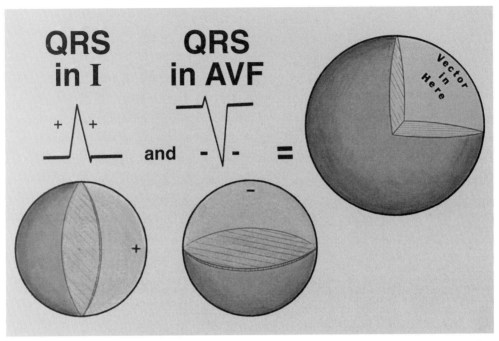

If the QRS is *positive* in lead I, and *negative* in AVF, that places the Vector in the upper left quadrant.

If the QRS in lead I is upright, the Vector points to the patient's _____.

left

If the Vector is pointing upward, then the QRS in lead AVF is mainly _____ the baseline.

below

And when the Vector points upward and to the patient's left, this is Left _____ Deviation (L.A.D.).

Axis

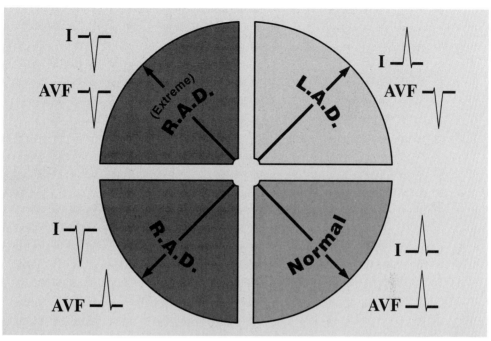

Now, by looking at the QRS complex in I and AVF, you can locate the Mean QRS Vector in an Axis quadrant (in the frontal plane as it relates to the patient).

Any time the QRS complex is negative in lead I, there is
_____ Axis Deviation (R.A.D.); and when the Vector   Right
also points upward (and to the patient's right), this is commonly
called "Extreme" R.A.D.

But if the QRS is positive in lead I and negative in lead AVF,
there is Left Axis _____.   Deviation

So if the Mean QRS Vector points downward and to the patient's left,
we expect the QRS complexes in leads I and AVF to be
mainly _____ (upright). And of course, they usually are,   positive
since this is normal.

NOTE: You also can calculate the vector for a portion of a QRS complex
(for instance, the initial or terminal .04 sec.) in exactly the same manner
as for the Mean QRS Vector.

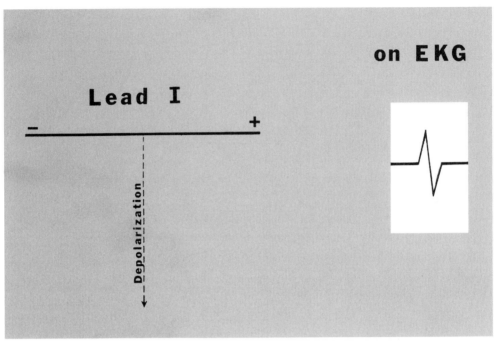

When depolarization moves in a direction perpendicular to the orientation of a lead, the deflection is minimal and/or "isoelectric". An isoelectric QRS records equal amounts of upward (positive) and negative (downward) deflection.

Depolarization that moves perpendicular to the orientation of a lead, is directed negligibly toward either electrode so the recorded deflection is as much negative as positive and is called _____.   isoelectric

The word "isoelectric" literally means "same voltage," so it is used when the positive and the negative portions of the QRS complex are about _____.   equal

Although the positive and negative deflections of an isoelectric QRS are equal in amplitude, they are generally small in the limb _____.   leads

NOTE: First, locate the Mean QRS Vector in an axis quadrant (i.e.; Normal, L.A.D., R.A.D., or Extreme R.A.D.). Then, find the limb lead in which the QRS is the most isoelectric, so you can more precisely locate the Vector in degrees (Axis). The Axis is about 90° from the orientation of the most isoelectric lead. It is really very easy...next page.

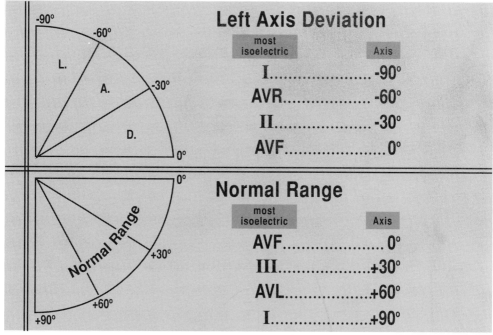

Left Axis Deviation

most isoelectric	Axis
I......................	-90°
AVR.................	-60°
II.....................	-30°
AVF...................	0°

Normal Range

most isoelectric	Axis
AVF....................	0°
III....................	+30°
AVL..................	+60°
I.....................	+90°

To locate the position of the Vector (Axis) more precisely (i.e., in degrees) in the frontal plane: <u>first</u> locate the axis quadrant, and <u>then</u> note the <u>limb</u> <u>lead</u> in which the QRS is most isoelectric.

NOTE: Please <u>refer to the illustration</u> on this page (and the page that follows) to determine the exact position of the Mean QRS Vector (Axis) in degrees. For exams and in "real life" situations you need a reference. Accuracy is far more important than memory. You may copy page 316; it's yours for real life use.

NOTE: Let's review. First, locate the appropriate axis quadrant. Then, to determine the exact position of the Vector (Axis), find the lead where the QRS is most isoelectric. Refer to the illustration as you contemplate the hypothetical examples below.

A patient with Left Axis Deviation has a Mean QRS Vector of between 0 and____ degrees (QRS positive in I and negative in AVF). Check the illustration.

-90
(don't forget the negative)

A young lady has a Mean QRS Vector in the normal range. If the QRS in lead III is isoelectric, then she has an electrical axis of ____. Please don't proceed to the next page until you feel comfortable with this exercise.

+30°

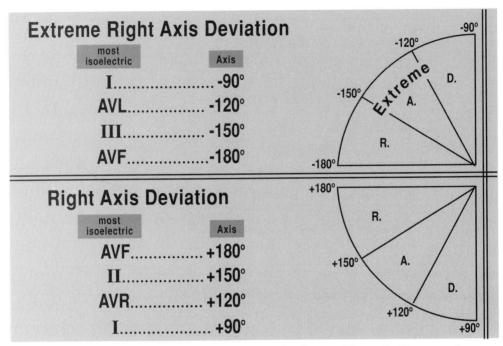

Extreme Right Axis Deviation

most isoelectric	Axis
I	-90°
AVL	-120°
III	-150°
AVF	-180°

Right Axis Deviation

most isoelectric	Axis
AVF	+180°
II	+150°
AVR	+120°
I	+90°

The exact position of the Vector (Axis) can be located in a similar way for Right Axis Deviation and Extreme Right Axis Deviation.

NOTE: After the axis quadrant is determined, the limb lead with the most isoelectric QRS is noted.*

Consider a patient with R.A.D. You find that the QRS is isoelectric in lead II, so the Axis is ____. See illustration to determine the answer for this blank and for those below.   +150°

You have a patient with numerous widened, premature QRS's, and you need to know whether it is a PVC or an aberrant Junctional beat. The wide QRS is negative in I and AVF, which places its Vector in the Extreme ____ quadrant (how could that be?)...   R.A.D.
...the wide QRS is also isoelectric in AVL, so its Axis is ____. For ventricular depolarization to progress in that direction,   -120°
it must have originated in a focus at the apex of the left ventricle, rather than from a Junctional focus. Let's think about that.

NOTE: An Axis of 180° is either + or - depending on whether the Vector is in the R.A.D. or Extreme R.A.D. quadrant respectively.

*This is summarized for you (page 316) of your **Personal Quick Reference Sheet**.

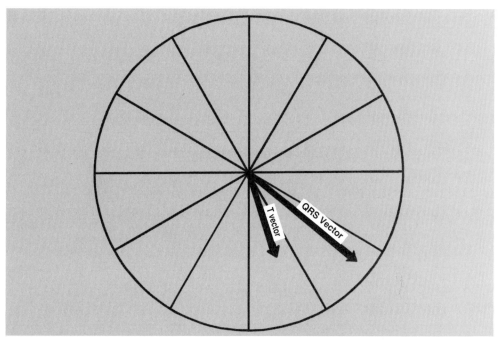

The Axis is sometimes depicted as the hands of a clock, the longer arrow is the Mean QRS Vector, the shorter is the T wave vector.

The T wave has a vector that can be located by using the same method used to locate the Mean _____ Vector in the frontal plane.   QRS

NOTE: When the T wave vector and the QRS Vector are separated by 60 degrees or more, this may signify pathology.

The T wave vector is usually represented as a smaller _____ than the QRS Vector.   arrow

NOTE: Axis is often denoted in medical literature by an "A" as in "A+30°" or "A = 30°", and it may be called "electrical axis."

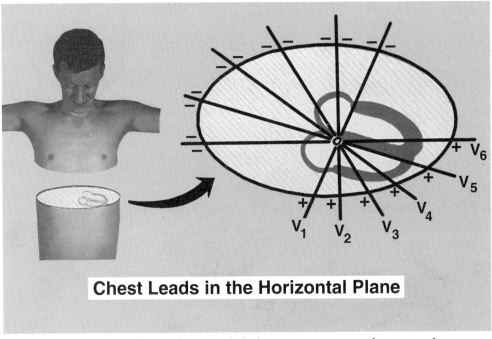

Chest Leads in the Horizontal Plane

The sphere has three dimensions, so it is important to note the general position of the Mean QRS Vector in the *horizontal* plane as well.

The horizontal _____ divides the body into top and bottom halves.

plane

The chest leads form the _____ plane.

horizontal

NOTE: To determine changes ("rotation") of the Mean QRS Vector in the <u>horizontal plane</u>, we examine the <u>chest leads</u>.

NOTE: Although the Axis may "deviate" in the frontal plane, the Vector is said to "rotate" in the horizontal plane. This is conventional (universally accepted) terminology used in communication and in medical literature.

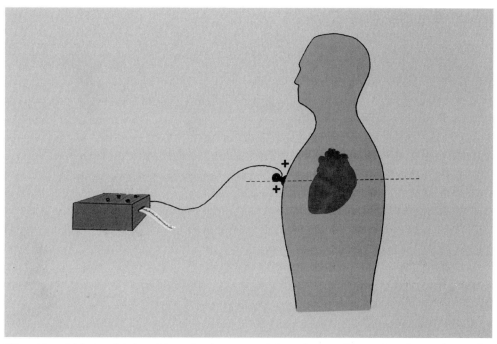

Chest lead V_2 is obtained by placing a positive electrode on the chest along the left side of the sternum (at the fourth interspace).

The chest electrode used for recording lead V_2 is always _____ (positive or negative).   positive

NOTE: The electrode for the chest leads is a suction cup that is moved to a different position on the chest for each of the six chest leads (which form the horizontal plane). In each case the suction cup electrode is positive.

The position of the (suction cup) electrode for recording lead V_2 places it in front of the heart at the fourth interspace to the left of the sternum, so it is just _____ to the AV Node.   anterior

NOTE: We already know that metal electrodes affixed with conductive gel are often used for recording the chest leads, so let's refocus on the conceptual material.

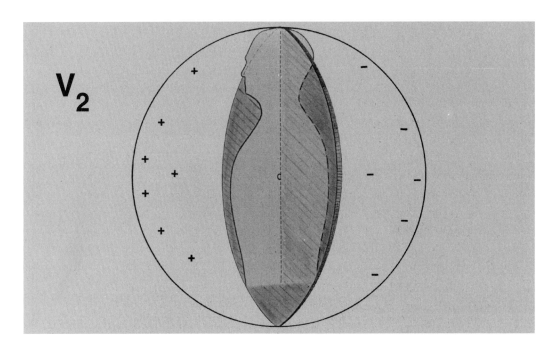

Considering the sphere for lead V_2 we can see that the front half is positive and the back half is negative.

Considering a lead V_2 sphere, we view the patient from the side. The center of the _____ is still the AV Node.

sphere

The patient's back is _____ (negative or positive), when considering lead V_2.

negative

The front half of the sphere is _____ in lead V_2.

positive

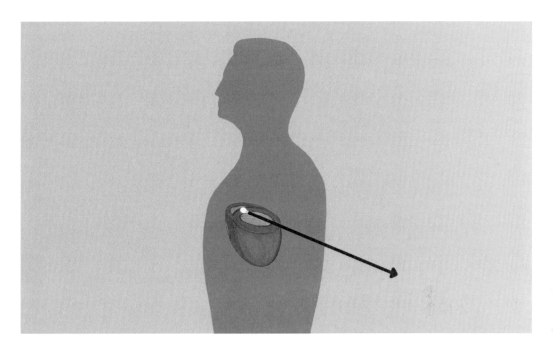

Normally the QRS in lead V₂ is negative. Therefore, the Mean QRS Vector points backward, because of the (generally) posterior position of the thick left ventricle.

Considering lead V₂ on the standard EKG, the QRS
complex is usually _____ (below the baseline).   negative

Therefore, the Mean QRS Vector usually points
_____ into the negative half of the sphere.   backward
                                                                      (posteriorly)

Normally, most of the ventricular depolarization is directed
away from the positive V₂ electrode, toward the thicker
and more posteriorly positioned ____ ventricle.   left

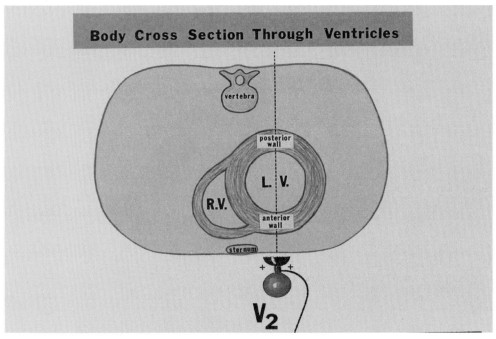

Body Cross Section Through Ventricles

vertebra

posterior wall

L. V.

R.V.

anterior wall

sternum

V₂

The orientation of chest lead V₂ makes it the most informative lead for the determination of both Anterior and Posterior Infarction.

The orientation of lead V₂ projects through the anterior wall
and the posterior wall of the _____ ventricle.   left

So V₂ reflects the most reliable information concerning Anterior
Infarction and _____ Infarction of the left ventricle.   Posterior

NOTE: As you will soon see, both ventricular depolarization
and repolarization should be scrutinized in the right chest leads,
because they reveal subtle vector changes caused by both anterior
and posterior infarctions (of the left ventricle).

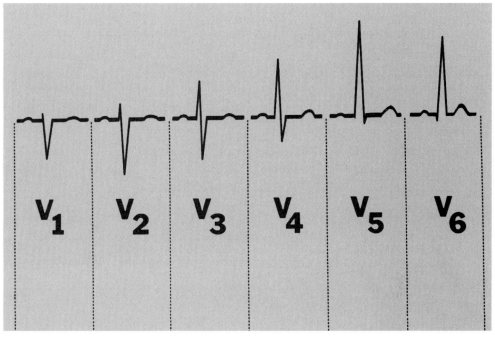

In the chest leads, there is a gradual transition from the generally negative QRS in V$_1$ to the generally positive (upright) QRS in V$_6$.

The QRS is mainly negative in lead V$_1$ and mostly
_____ in lead V$_6$.   positive

Examining chest leads V$_1$ through V$_6$ to observe the gradual
transition of QRS complexes, we notice that the QRS usually
becomes as much positive as negative or "_____"   isoelectric
in lead V$_3$ or V$_4$. This is the *transitional zone*.

NOTE: You will recall that an isoelectric QRS is 90° away from
the Mean QRS Vector. So a shift ("rotation") of the Vector in the
horizontal plane is reflected as a similar change in position of the
"transitional" (isoelectric) QRS in the chest leads. You will better
understand and appreciate this when you see the next page.

As the Vector changes its position (rotates) in the horizontal plane,
the Vector's tail remains anchored to the ___ _____.   AV Node

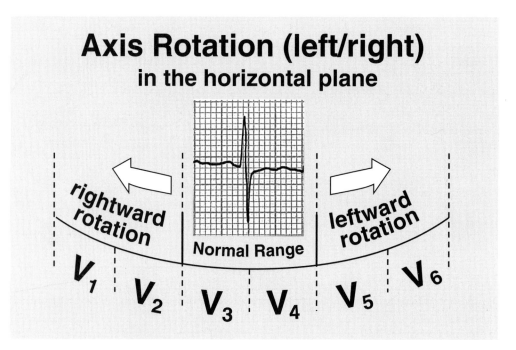

Axis Rotation (left/right)
in the horizontal plane

Rotation of the Vector in the horizontal plane is described from the patient's point of view as "rightward" or "leftward". Check the chest leads for the isoelectric QRS.

NOTE: The Vector can *rotate* in the horizontal plane with its tail anchored to the AV Node. When the isoelectric ("transitional") QRS has rotated to the patient's right (into leads V_1 or V_2) this is *rightward* rotation. But if the transitional QRS is found in the patient's left chest leads, V_5 or V_6 this is *leftward* rotation. Anatomically speaking the heart is not capable of much rotation in the horizontal plane. But we do know that the Vector shifts toward Ventricular Hypertrophy and away from Infarction.

NOTE: In older literature you may still see the terms "clockwise" (meaning leftward) rotation or "counterclockwise" (meaning rightward) rotation of the Vector in the horizontal plane. These terms have become obsolete since they do not relate well to clocks, and much confusion resulted.

REMINDER: Axis deviation is in the frontal plane.
                    Axis rotation is in the horizontal plane.

NOTE: Please observe the simplified technique for determining Axis by turning to page 310. A quick review of the methodology may be found in the **P**ersonal **Q**uick **R**eference **S**heets on page 316.

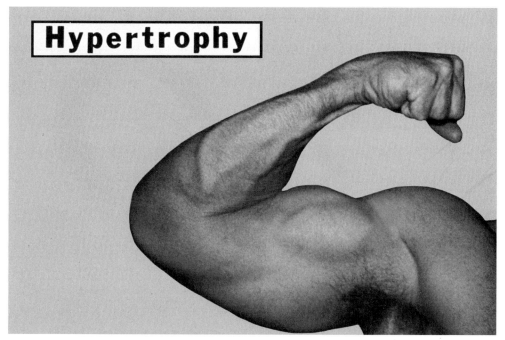

Hypertrophy usually pertains to an increase in size, but when relating to muscle as in myocardium, this term refers to increase in muscle mass.

NOTE: The photo above is the arm of a weight lifter. I had contemplated using a photo of my own arm, but I soon abandoned the idea because then I would have to title this section "hypotrophy" (if there is such a word).

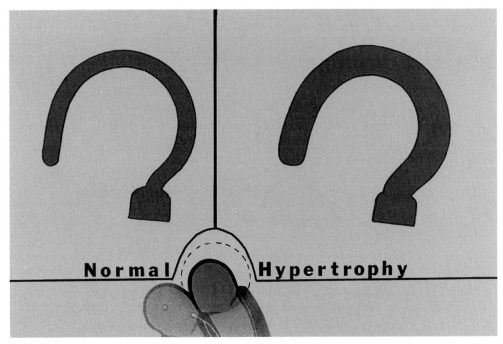

Normal   Hypertrophy

Hypertrophy of a chamber of the heart implies an increase in the thickness of the chamber wall, but some dilation is always present also.

Hypertrophy of a chamber of the heart means that the muscular wall of that chamber has dilated and thickened beyond _____ thickness.

normal

Hypertrophy may increase the volume that the _____ contains, and the wall of that chamber is thicker than normal.

chamber

The increase in the muscular thickness of the wall of a hypertrophic chamber, as well as dilation of a chamber of the heart may be diagnosed on _____.

EKG

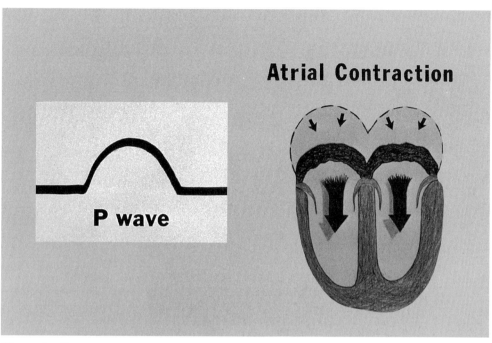

Since the P wave represents the depolarization and contraction of both atria, we examine the P wave for evidence of atrial enlargement.

The depolarization of both atria causes their simultaneous
_____.

contraction

The depolarization of both atria is recorded on EKG as
a ___ wave.

P

Signs of atrial enlargement can be detected by examining
the P wave on the twelve lead _____.

EKG

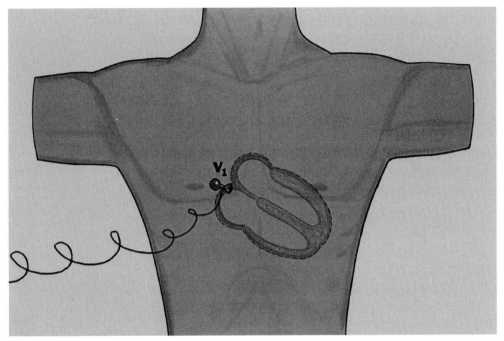

Lead V_1 is directly over the atria, so the P wave in V_1 is our best source of information about atrial enlargement (see NOTE).

(free   P₃ 50)

The chest electrode that records lead V_1 is considered
_____ (positive or negative).   positive

When lead V_1 is recording, the electrode is positioned just
to the right of the sternum in the 4th interspace; this places
the electrode directly over the _____.   atria

Because the V_1 electrode is close to the atria, the P wave
in lead V_1 gives us the most accurate information about
atrial _____.   enlargement
                                                                           (see NOTE)

NOTE: Since the atria dilate more than they hypertrophy, physicians refer to
"atrial enlargement." Whereas when referring to the ventricles, "ventricular
hypertrophy" predominates.

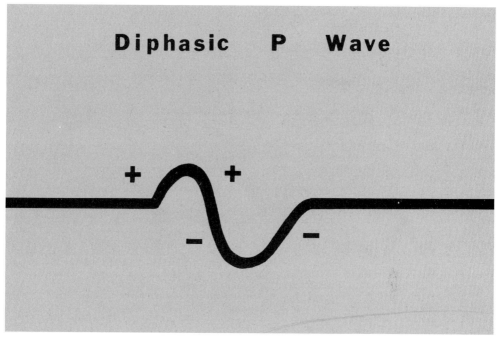

With atrial enlargement, the P wave is usually *diphasic* (both positive and negative).

A wave which has both positive and negative portions is called a _____ wave (two phased wave).   diphasic

A diphasic P wave has deflections above and below the _____.   baseline

The diphasic P wave is characteristic of atrial enlargement, but we want to know which of the two _____ is enlarged.   atria

Right Atrial Hypertrophy

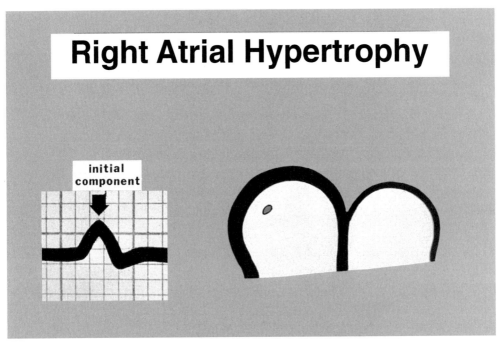

initial component

If the initial component of a diphasic P wave (in lead V$_1$) is the larger, then this is *Right Atrial Enlargement.*

If the P wave in lead V$_1$ is _____, then we know that one of the atria is enlarged.

diphasic

If the initial portion of the diphasic P wave is the _____ of the two phases, then there is Right Atrial Enlargement.

larger

A diphasic P wave in V$_1$ with a large, often peaked, initial component tells us that this patient's _____ atrium is probably thicker and more dilated than his left.

right

NOTE: If the height of the P wave in any of the limb leads exceeds 2.5 mm (even if it's not diphasic), suspect Right Atrial Enlargement.

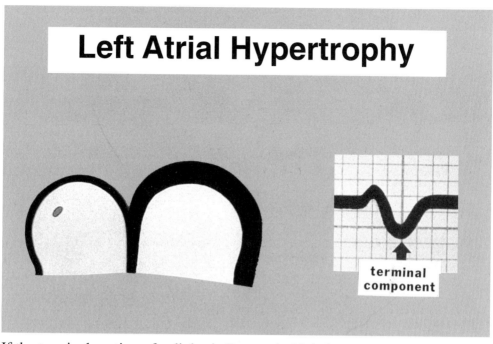

Left Atrial Hypertrophy

terminal
component

If the terminal portion of a diphasic P wave in V$_1$ is large and wide, there is *Left Atrial Enlargement*.

A patient who has enlargement of the left atrium, because the mitral valve is stenosed*, will have a diphasic P wave in lead ___ .

V$_1$

This patient's diphasic P wave in lead V$_1$ has a small initial component and a larger _____ component.

terminal

The terminal component of a diphasic P wave in lead V$_1$ is usually _____ (positive or negative).

negative

*A narrowed mitral valve can cause left atrial enlargement, but systemic hypertension is the most common cause.

235

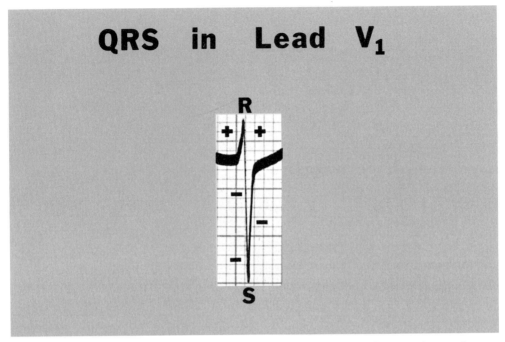

Now let's consider the QRS complex in V₁. Normally the S wave is much larger than the R wave in this lead.

The QRS complex represents ventricular depolarization, so we would expect the QRS to reflect some indications of the presence of ventricular _____.   hypertrophy

In lead V₁ the QRS complex is mainly _____,   negative
and therefore the R wave is usually very short.

NOTE: The V₁ electrode is positive. Ventricular depolarization moves downward to the patient's left side and also posteriorly (the thicker left ventricle is more posteriorly located). Because ventricular depolarization is moving AWAY from the (positive) V₁ electrode, the QRS in V₁ is usually mainly negative. Remember that the positive wave of depolarization moving toward a positive electrode records a positive deflection on EKG. By the same token, depolarization moving away from a positive electrode records negatively.

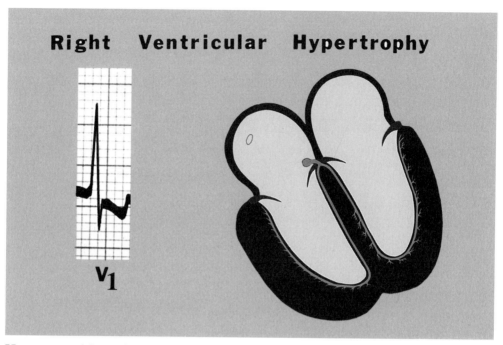

Right Ventricular Hypertrophy

V_1

However, with *Right Ventricular Hypertrophy* (RVH) there is a large R wave in V_1.

In Right Ventricular Hypertrophy there is a large ____ wave in lead V_1.

R

NOTE: With Right Ventricular Hypertrophy, the wall of the right ventricle is very thick, so there is much more (positive) depolarization (and more vectors) toward the (positive) V_1 electrode. We would therefore expect the QRS in lead V_1 to be more positive (upright) than usual.

The S wave in lead V_1 is smaller than the ____ wave in Right Ventricular Hypertrophy. (See illustration).

R

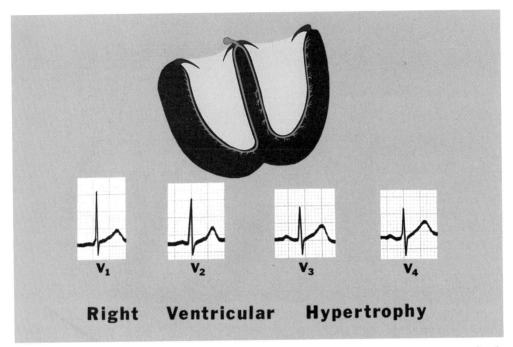

Right   Ventricular   Hypertrophy

With Right Ventricular Hypertrophy, the large R wave of V_1 gets progressively smaller from V_2 to V_3 to V_4 etc.

When Right Ventricular Hypertrophy is present, there is a large R wave in lead ___ that becomes progressively smaller in chest leads V_2, V_3, and V_4.

V_1

The progressive decrease in the height of the ___ wave is gradual, proceeding from the right chest leads to the left chest leads.

R

NOTE: The enlarged right ventricle adds more vectors toward the right side, so there is Right Axis Deviation (in the frontal plane), and in the horizontal plane there is rightward rotation of the (Mean QRS) Vector. Visualize the reasons for these (Mean QRS) Vector shifts and the criteria will become very logical.

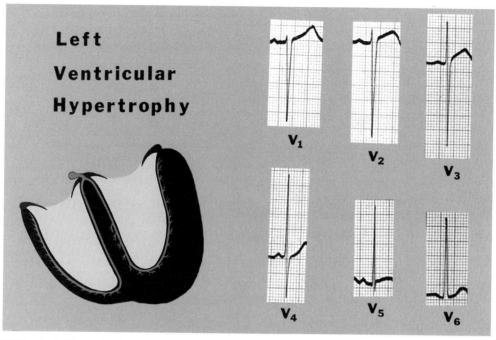

With *Left Ventricular Hypertrophy* (LVH), the left ventricular wall is very thick, causing great QRS deflections in the chest leads.

The heart chamber with the thickest muscular walls
is the _____ ventricle.

left

Hypertrophy of the left ventricle produces QRS complexes
that are exaggerated amplitude, both in height and in depth,
especially in the _____ leads.

chest

NOTE: Normally the S wave in V_1 is deep. But with Left Ventricular
Hypertrophy even more depolarization is going downward to the patient's
left – away from the positive V_1 electrode. Therefore the S wave
is even deeper in V_1. There is Left Axis Deviation, and often
the Vector is displaced in a leftward direction in the horizontal plane.
Visualize and understand the reason for these shifts of the Vector.
Lasting knowledge results from understanding.

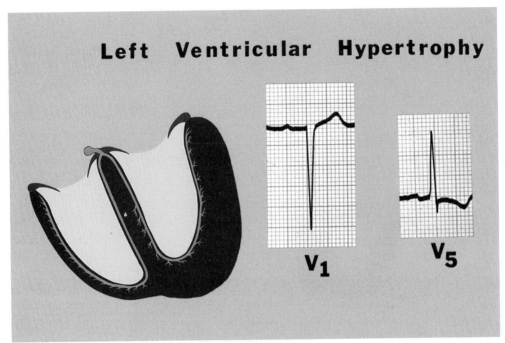

Left Ventricular Hypertrophy

V₁   V₅

With Left Ventricular Hypertrophy there is a large S in V_1 and a large R in V_5.

With Left Ventricular Hypertrophy there is a very tall ____
wave in lead V_5 .

R

NOTE: Lead V_5 is over the left ventricle, so the increased
depolarization is going toward the electrode of V_5 when
there is L.V.H. This results in more (positive) depolarization
going toward the (positive) electrode of V_5 which produces a
very tall R wave in that lead.

In Left Ventricular Hypertrophy there is a very tall R wave
in lead ___, and this excessive depolarization moving away
from the V_1 electrode produces a deep S wave in lead V_1 .

V_5

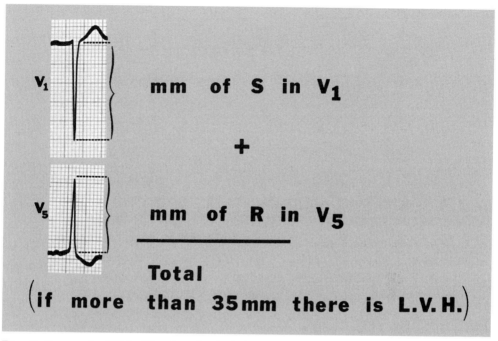

mm of S in V$_1$

+

mm of R in V$_5$

_____

Total

(if more than 35mm there is L.V.H.)

Depth (in mm) of S in V$_1$ plus the height of R in V$_5$ . . . if greater than 35 mm, there is Left Ventricular Hypertrophy.

To check an EKG for Left Ventricular Hypertrophy, just add the depth of the S wave in V$_1$ to the height of the____ wave in V$_5$.

R

If the depth (in mm) of the S wave in V$_1$ added to the height (in mm) of the R wave in V$_5$ is greater than 35 (mm), then _____ Ventricular Hypertrophy is present.

Left

NOTE: The sum of the S in V$_1$ plus the R in V$_5$ should be routinely checked (mere observation will usually suffice) with every twelve lead EKG. When providing a written EKG interpretation, however, one should measure and document the amplitude of these waves in millimeters.

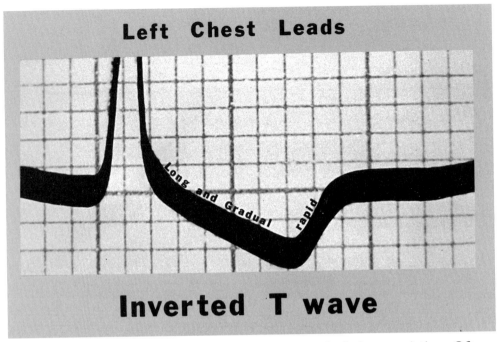

Left Chest Leads

Long and Gradual rapid

Inverted T wave

The T wave may show "Left Ventricular Hypertrophy" characteristics. Often there is T wave *inversion* with T wave *asymmetry*.

There is a characteristic T wave that is commonly associated with _____ Ventricular Hypertrophy.

Left

Since the left chest leads (V_5 or V_6) are over the left _____, these are ideal leads to check for this characteristic T wave that we find with LVH.

ventricle

With LVH, the *inverted* T wave has a gradual downslope and a very steep return to the _____, making it *asymmetrical*.

baseline

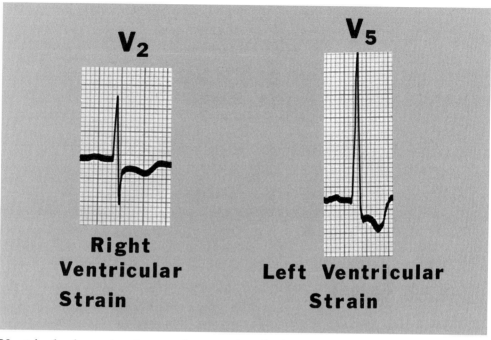

Ventricular hypertrophy may be associated with a *strain* pattern. With *ventricular strain* the ST segment becomes depressed and humped.

Ventricular strain is characterized by depression of the
ST _____.   segment

NOTE: Strain is usually associated with ventricular hypertrophy, which is logical, since a ventricle that is straining against some kind of resistance (e.g., increased resistance from a narrowed valve or from hypertension) will become hypertrophied in its attempt to compensate.

Ventricular strain causes a depressed ST segment, which generally humps upward in the middle of the _____.   segment

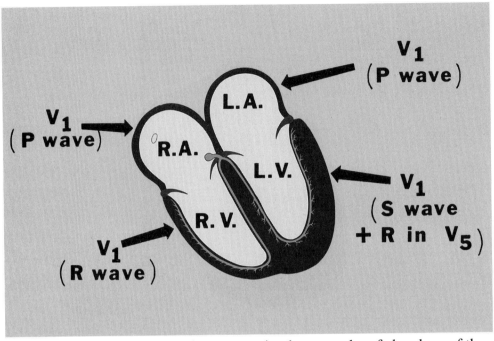

Note that most of the information concerning hypertrophy of chambers of the heart is provided in lead V_1.

When routinely reading a 12 lead EKG, you should check to see if there is _____ of any of the chambers.

hypertrophy

First, check lead V_1 to see if the P waves are _____.

diphasic

Second, check the R wave in V_1 . . . and then check the S wave in V_1 and the ___ wave in V_5.

R

NOTE: You may now review Hypertrophy by turning to the **Personal Quick Reference** Sheets on page 317, and relate this to the simplified methodology that is summarized on page 310.

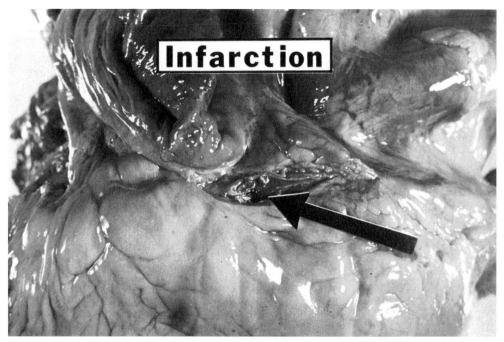

Myocardial Infarction (M.I.) results from the complete occlusion of a coronary artery. The area of myocardium supplied by the occluded coronary artery becomes non-viable and neither depolarizes nor contracts.

NOTE: Although the heart's chambers are filled with blood, the myocardium's own blood supply is provided exclusively by the coronary arteries. A coronary artery can be gradually narrowed by lipid deposits that become *atheromatous plaque* beneath the intimal lining of the vessel. The *intima* may eventually rupture, exposing the plaque to the blood within the artery. This initiates the immediate formation of a clot (*thrombus*). The vessel, already narrowed by the plaque, becomes totally occluded by the thrombus. Instantly an area of the heart is without blood supply and is devoid of function...worse yet, the resulting cardiac hypoxia can cause marked irritability in one or more ventricular foci, producing a deadly arrhythmia.

NOTE: Myocardial Infarction implies the complete occlusion of a coronary artery, which we can diagnose with the EKG. The electrocardiogram will also tell us which coronary artery (or coronary branch) is occluded, and it can even reveal any blocks in the ventricular conduction caused by the infarction. By careful interpretation of the EKG we can also determine if a coronary vessel is narrowed rendering a decreased blood supply to the heart. Practical lifesaving knowledge. Let me show you...

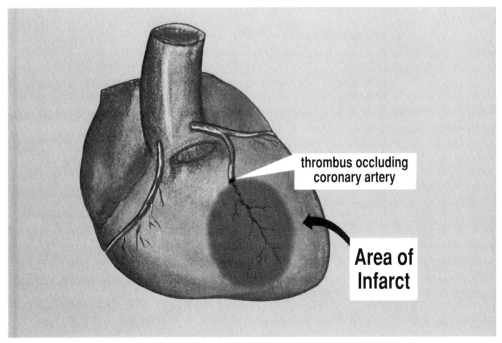

thrombus occluding
coronary artery

**Area of
Infarct**

Myocardial infarction occurs when a coronary artery supplying the left ventricle becomes occluded, so an area of the heart* is without a blood supply.

The terms "myocardial _____," "coronary occlusion," and "heart attack" refer to the same serious phenomenon.   infarction

The heart derives its own blood supply from the _____   coronary
arteries, so when a coronary artery or one of its major branches
is occluded, an area of the myocardium is without blood supply.

The infarcted area is primarily in the _____ ventricle, and   left
deadly arrhythmias may result.

NOTE: We understand that the coronary arteries also supply the
right ventricle, so there is often some involvement of the right ventricle.
But since most of the critical problems originate in left ventricular infarcts,
myocardial infarction is usually conceptualized in terms of the left ventricle.

* In this illustration, the pulmonary artery has been "surgically" removed to show the origin of
  the coronary arteries at the base of the aorta.

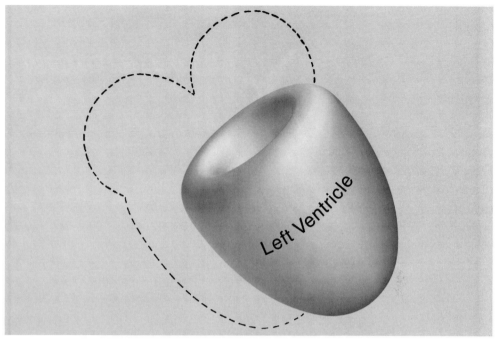

Commonly, the thick left ventricle suffers myocardial infarction.

The left ventricle is the thickest chamber of the heart; so if
the coronary arteries are narrowed, the left ventricle (which
uses the greatest blood supply) is the first to suffer from
an obstructed coronary _____.   artery

Blood is pumped to all parts of the body by the powerful,
thick, _____ ventricle.   left

NOTE: When we describe infarcts by location, we are speaking
of an area within the left ventricle. Coronary arteries to the left
ventricle usually send smaller branches to other regions of the heart,
so an infarction of the left ventricle can include a small portion of
another chamber.

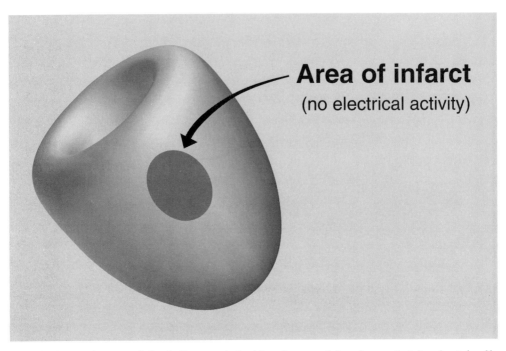

Area of infarct
(no electrical activity)

This infarcted area of the left ventricle (that has no blood supply) is electrically dead and cannot conduct depolarization.

Infarctions usually involve an area of the wall of the left _____.

ventricle

An area of infarction cannot be depolarized because the cells there are without a _____ supply, and they are functionally dead.

blood

NOTE: This infarcted area produces an electrical void, while the rest of the heart (with an adequate blood supply) functions as usual. The infarcted region does not depolarize, so it does not contract, thereby impairing the muscular function of the left ventricle.

Ischemia

Injury

Infarction

The classic triad of a myocardial infarction is "ISCHEMIA," "INJURY," and "INFARCTION," but any of the three may occur alone.

The "three I" triad is the basis for recognizing and diagnosing
_____ infarction.   myocardial

The word *hypoxia* means decreased oxygen; in the heart it
is usually caused by *ischemia,* which literally means reduced
_____ supply (diminished blood flow).   blood

NOTE: Ischemia, Injury, and Infarction need not all be present
at once in order to establish the diagnosis of myocardial infarction.
The three I triad is a memory tool of routine criteria to check for
myocardial infarction.

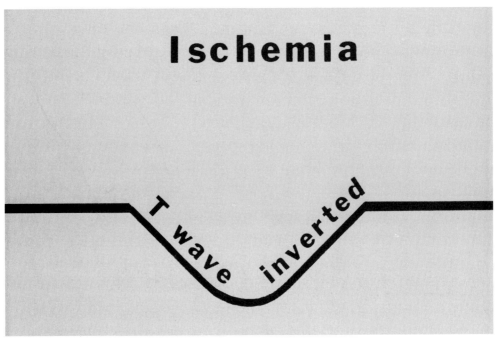

Ischemia (decreased blood supply) is characterized by inverted T waves.

↳ may Result in Peaked T Waves. (See below)

Ischemia means reduced _____ supply (from the coronary arteries) or less than is normally present.

blood

The characteristic sign of ischemia is the _____ T wave. It may vary from a slightly inverted to a deeply inverted T wave.

inverted

Inverted ___ waves may indicate ischemia in the absence of myocardial infarction. Coronary blood flow can be diminished without producing an infarction.

T

Formi: Current Med Dx lists classic evolution of EKG changes as Peaked "hyper Acute" T waves, to ST seg elevation, + Q wave, to T-wave Inversion.

Ischemia

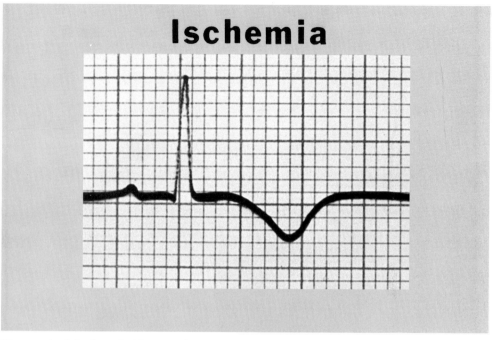

The typical ischemia T wave is symmetrically inverted.

NOTE: You should check every EKG that you read for T wave inversion. Since the chest leads are nearest the ventricles, T wave changes are most pronounced in these leads. Always run down V_1 to V_6 (as well as the limb leads) and check for T wave inversion to see if there is diminished coronary flow.

The T wave of ischemia is inverted, and it is _____; that is, the right and left sides of the inverted T wave are mirror images.

symmetrical

NOTE: In adults flat (nonexistent) T waves or minimal T wave inversion may be a normal variant in any of the limb leads (frontal plane). However, any T wave inversion in leads V_2 through V_6 is considered pathological.

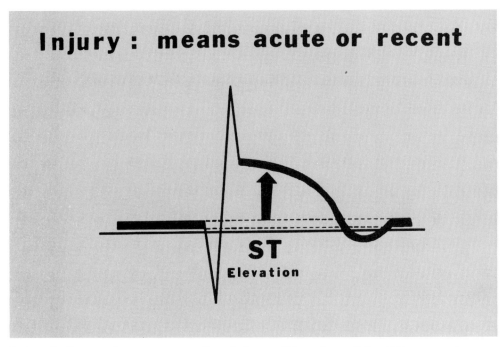

Injury : means acute or recent

ST
Elevation

Injury indicates the acuteness of an infarct. Elevation of the ST segment denotes "injury."

NOTE: "Acute" means recent.

The ST segment is that section of baseline between the
QRS complex and the ___ wave. The ST segment   T
contains no waves.

Elevation of the ___ segment signifies "injury." The   ST
ST segment may be only slightly elevated, or as much
as ten or more millimeters above the baseline.

ST segment elevation tells us that a myocardial
infarction is _____. It is the earliest sign of infarction   acute
to record on EKG.

ST Elevation

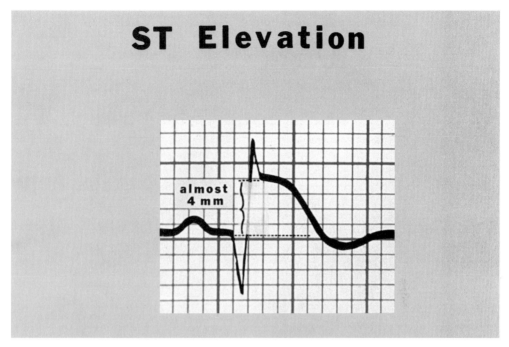

almost
4 mm

If there is ST elevation, this indicates that the infarction is acute. ST elevation, alone, can indicate an infarction.

NOTE: Once you have made a diagnosis of infarction, it is important to know whether the infarction just occurred and needs immediate treatment, or if the infarction is old — maybe years old.

The ST _____ rises above the baseline with an acute   segment infarction, in fact it is usually the earliest EKG sign of an infarction. With time, the ST segment returns to the baseline.

NOTE: If the ST segment is elevated without associated Q waves, this may represent *non-Q wave infarction*, which is usually a small infarction that may herald an impending larger infarct. Significant ST changes require enzyme studies and close scrutiny.

NOTE: A *ventricular aneurysm* (the outward ballooning of the wall of a ventricle) may also cause ST elevation, but the ST segment in this case does *not* return to the baseline with time. *Pericarditis* (next page) produces a unique type of ST segment elevation that may also elevate the T wave off the baseline.

Pericarditis

flat or concave elevated ST segment | **elevated ST segment and T wave off baseline**

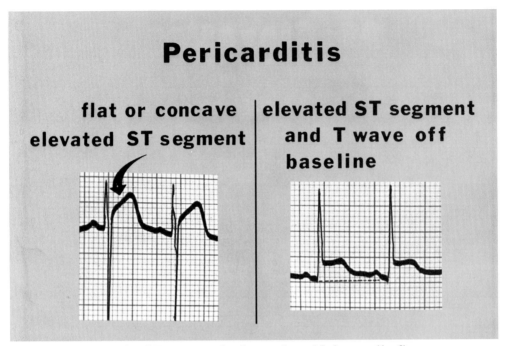

With *pericarditis* the ST segment is elevated, and it is usually flat or concave. The entire T wave may be elevated off the baseline.

NOTE: Pericarditis is inflammation of the fluid-filled sac (*pericardium*) that surrounds the heart. Pericarditis may be caused by a virus, bacteria, cancer, or other sources of inflammation, including myocardial infarction.

Pericarditis can elevate the ___ segment. It usually produces an elevated ST segment that is flat or slightly concave (middle sags downward). This resolves with time.

ST

Pericarditis seems to elevate the entire ___ wave off the baseline; that is, the baseline gradually angles back down (often including the P wave) all the way to the next QRS (illustration on right).

T

NOTE: The characteristics shown in the left illustration are found in a lead in which the QRS is usually mainly negative (like the right chest leads). The pattern shown in the right illustration is seen in leads where the QRS is mainly positive (such as leads I or II).

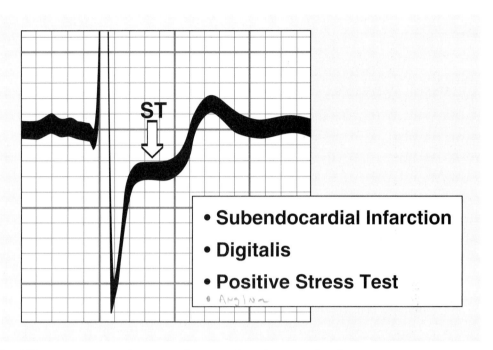

- **Subendocardial Infarction**
- **Digitalis**
- **Positive Stress Test**
  ● Angina

The ST segment may become depressed under certain circumstances or conditions.

NOTE: During an angina* attack the ST segment may be temporarily depressed.

Digitalis can cause _____ of the ST segment, however it has a unique, unforgettable appearance (see page 296).   depression

When a patient with narrowed coronaries exercises, the myocardium demands more blood flow than its arteries can deliver. A *Stress* (or "Exercise") *Test* will record depression of the ___ segment on EKG when such a patient is exercised.   ST

A subendocardial infarction — an infarct that does not extend through the full thickness of the _____ ventricular wall — will depress the ST segment.   left

*Chest pain caused by diminished coronary blood flow.

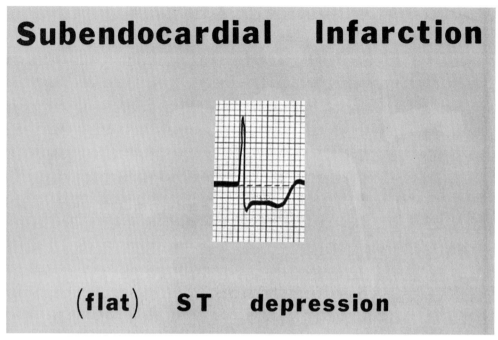

Subendocardial Infarction

(flat) ST depression

Subendocardial infarction causes a flat depression of the ST segment; however, any significant ST depression indicates compromised coronary blood flow until proven otherwise.

Subendocardial infarction (often referred to as subendocardial injury) is identified by flat ST _____ depression, which segment may be either horizontal or down-sloping.

NOTE: Subendocardial infarction, a type of "non-Q wave infarction" involves only a small area of myocardium just beneath the endocardial lining. Classical myocardial infarction is said to be *transmural*; that is, the full thickness of the left ventricular wall is damaged in the infarcted area. Even though subendocardial infarction involves only a small area of the myocardium, it must be respected as a true M.I. that requires appropriate care. A subendocardial M.I. may enlarge or extend to become more life-threatening.

NOTE: Any patient with acute ST depression (or elevation), particularly if it persists, should have an immediate, complete workup including cardiac enzymes.

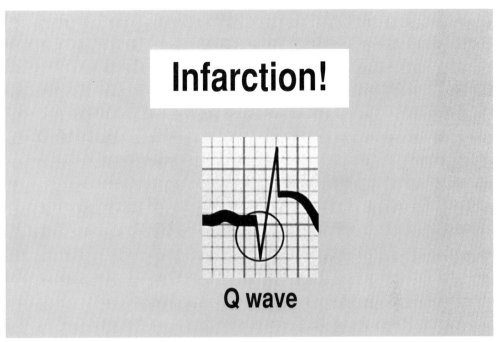

Infarction!

Q wave

The Q wave makes the diagnosis of infarction.

The diagnosis of myocardial infarction is usually based on the
presence of significant ___ waves.   Q

NOTE: The Q wave is the first downward stroke of the QRS complex,
and it is never preceded by anything in the complex. In the QRS complex,
if there is any positive wave — even a tiny spike — before the
downward wave, the downward is an S wave (and the upward wave
preceding it is an R wave).

Significant Q _____ are absent in normal tracings.   waves
We use a capital "Q" to designate a significant Q wave,
however "q" waves are not significant.

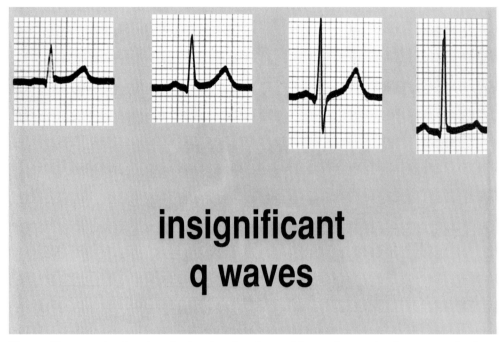

insignificant
q waves

Normally ventricular depolarization begins midway down the interventricular septum. Septal depolarization is left-to-right and this <u>initial</u> rightward ventricular activation may produce tiny, *insignificant q* (small q) *waves* in some leads.

The Right Bundle Branch traverses the septum without branching, however the _____ Bundle Branch gives off terminal Purkinje filaments at mid-septum.

Left

So this <u>initial</u> mid-septal depolarization moves left-to-right, away from:
- the positive left arm electrode of lateral leads I and AVL and...
- the positive chest electrode of left chest leads V_5 and V_6 and...
- somewhat away from the positive left foot electrode of leads II, III, and AVF...

... to occasionally record tiny, insignificant __ waves in those leads.

q

NOTE: This mid-septal depolarization is brief since the efficient ventricular conduction system quickly transmits depolarization to the endocardial surface of both ventricles. So brief is this mid-septal depolarization that only a tiny q wave of less than .04 second is recorded. Insignificant q waves are, by definition, less than one millimeter (.04 sec.) duration.

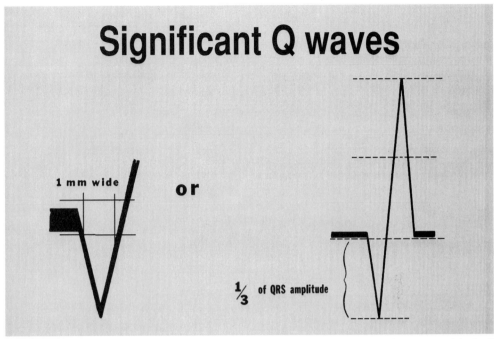

Significant Q waves

1 mm wide

or

⅓ of QRS amplitude

A *significant Q wave* is at least one small square wide (.04 sec.) or one-third of the entire QRS amplitude. Significant Q waves indicate a myocardial infarction.

Significant Q waves are indicative of pathology — namely the presence of a myocardial _____.

infarction

A significant Q wave is one small square (one millimeter) or more wide, and therefore is at least ___ second or more in duration.

.04

An old, but persistent, criterion of the significant Q wave is when the Q wave is _____ the amplitude (height and depth) of the entire QRS complex.

one-third

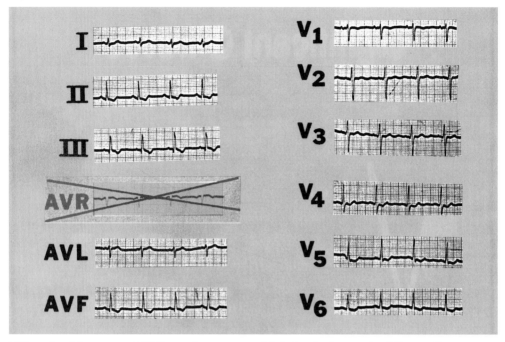

When looking at an EKG tracing, note which leads have significant Q waves. Omit lead AVR.

To check for an infarction we scan all leads for the presence of _____ Q waves.   significant

NOTE: Forget about lead AVR, since this lead is positioned in such a way that data regarding Q waves are unreliable. Lead AVR is like an upside-down lead II, so the large Q waves that are commonly seen in lead AVR are really the upside-down R waves from lead II. Even if you don't understand the logic behind AVR's phony Q's, don't bother to check it for signs of infarction.

When examining a tracing, either long strip or mounted, write down those _____ in which you find significant Q* waves,   leads
ST segment elevation (or depression), and inverted T waves.

*For proper documentation, insignificant q waves should be recorded as well.

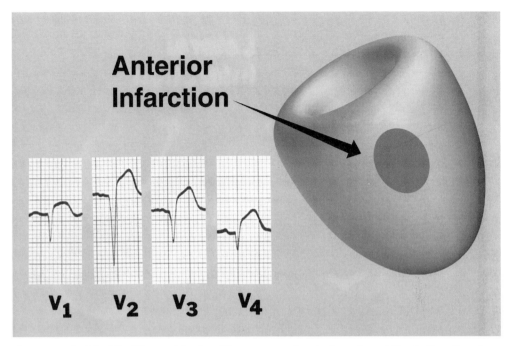

Q waves in V_1, V_2, V_3, or V_4 signify an *anterior infarction*. The infarction in the illustration is definitely acute, because of the ST elevation in all four leads.

NOTE: The chest leads are mainly placed anteriorly, so this is a good way to remember the leads for anterior infarction.

The presence of Q waves in V_1, V_2, V_3, or V_4 indicates an infarction in the anterior wall of the _____ ventricle.   left

NOTE: The anterior portion of the left ventricle includes part of the interventricular septum. Some cardiologists say that when isolated Q waves appear in V_1 and V_2, the infarction includes the septum, so it is called an antero-*septal* infarction. Similarly, isolated Q waves in V_3 and V_4 (more laterally located chest leads) are said to represent an antero-*lateral* infarction. Remember that (insignificant) q waves are seen normally in V_5 and V_6.

see ACLS Book

NOTE: Statistically, anterior infarctions are very deadly, but fortunately, immediate treatment with intravenous thrombolytic medications has improved the survival rate substantially.

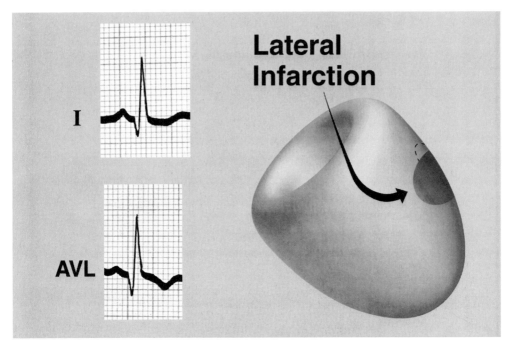

Lateral Infarction

If there are Q waves in lead I and lead AVL, there is a *lateral infarction.*

NOTE: Please take a moment and glance at page 46 to make a mental note of the leads that have a positive electrode located laterally on the left arm.

A lateral infarction involves the lateral portion of the _____ ventricle.   left

When a lateral infarction occurs, __ waves appear in   Q
leads I and AVL. The infarct illustrated above is old
(ST segments are at baseline level).

NOTE: One might abbreviate Lateral Infarction as L.I. Just remember
AV<u>L</u> for "Lateral" and "I" for Infarction (after all, Roman Numeral "I" is
just a capital "i"). It's an easy way to recall the leads that demonstrate lateral
infarction.

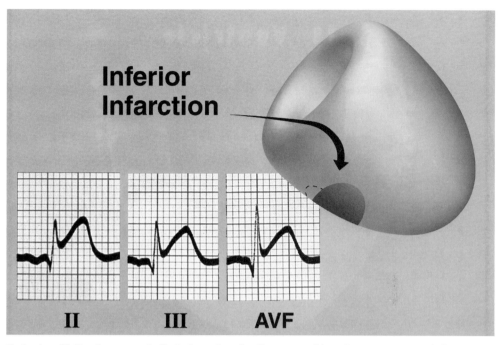

Inferior Infarction

II   III   AVF

Inferior ("diaphragmatic") *infarction* is diagnosed by the presence of Q waves in II, III, and AVF. Check the ST segments to see if this infarction is acute.

The inferior wall of the heart rests upon the diaphragm, so the term "diaphragmatic" infarction refers to an infarction in the inferior portion of the left _____.   ventricle

NOTE: Please return to page 46 to reinforce your knowledge concerning the leads that have a positive electrode located (inferiorly) on the left foot.

An _____ infarction is identified by significant Q waves   inferior
in leads II, III, and AVF.

NOTE: If I told you the way that I remember the leads for inferior infarction, this book would be banned. You may want to make your own memory tool for remembering the leads for Inferior ("diaphragmatic") Infarction using "two, three, and F."

NOTE: Autopsy data show that about one-third of inferior infarctions also include portions of the right ventricle.

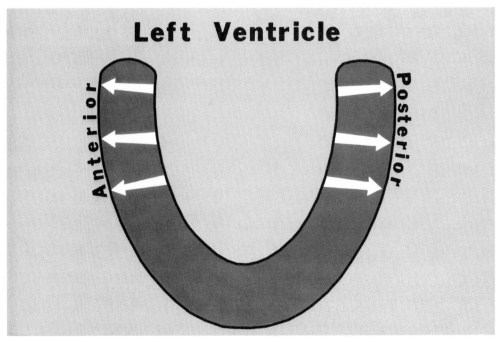

Notice that depolarization of the anterior wall and depolarization of the posterior wall of the left ventricle are in opposite directions.

NOTE: Left ventricular depolarization may be said to proceed from the *endocardium* (inner lining) to the *epicardium* (outer surface).

Depolarization of the anterior wall of the left ventricle proceeds from the inner endocardium, which lines the ventricle, through the full thickness of the ventricular wall to the outer ventricular surface (_____).   epicardium

Similarly, depolarization of the posterior wall of the _____   left
ventricle proceeds from the endocardium to the epicardium.

So vectors representing depolarization of the anterior and the posterior portions of the left ventricle point in _____ directions.   opposite

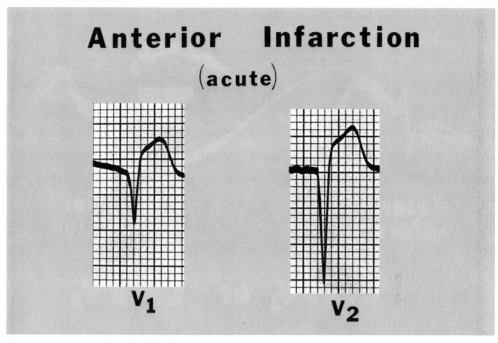

If an acute anterior infarction produces Q waves and ST elevation in V_1 and V_2 then a posterior infarction would appear the opposite.

An acute anterior infarction produces significant Q waves with ST _____ in the first few chest leads.

elevation

Considering only V_1 and V_2 the appearance of significant Q waves and ST elevation would indicate an acute _____ infarction.

anterior
(antero-septal)

NOTE: Acute posterior infarction of the left ventricle would produce the exact opposite to the pattern of acute anterior infarction, because the anterior and posterior walls of the left ventricle depolarize in opposite directions.

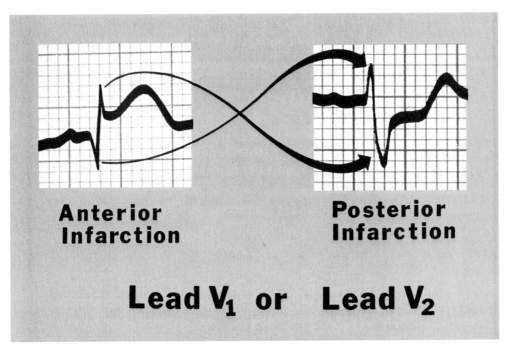

Anterior Infarction

Posterior Infarction

Lead V₁ or Lead V₂

In acute *Posterior Infarction* there is a large R wave (the opposite of a Q wave) in V_1 and V_2.

NOTE: In lead V_1 a Q wave turned upside-down would look like an R wave (and as you recall, R waves in lead V_1 are normally very tiny).

A significant "Q wave" from an infarction in the posterior portion of the _____ ventricle will cause a large R (positive deflection) wave to appear in lead V_1.

left

Suspect a true posterior infarction when you see a large __ wave in V_1 or V_2 — even though Right Ventricular Hypertrophy can also produce a large R in V_1.

R

266

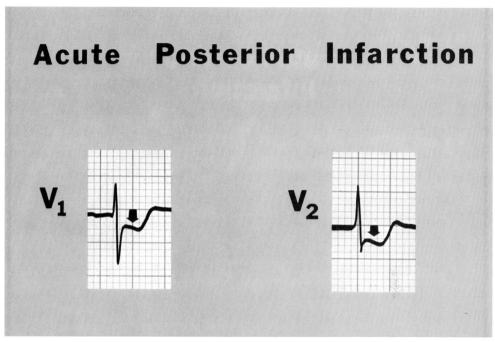

Acute   Posterior   Infarction

In acute posterior infarction, there is ST <u>depression</u> (the opposite of the usual ST elevation of Injury) in V_1 or V_2.

Acute anterior infarction produces Q waves in the chest leads and the ST segments are _____.   elevated

NOTE: Since the posterior wall of the left ventricle depolarizes in a direction opposite to that of the anterior wall, an acute infarction of the posterior wall causes ST DEPRESSION in V_1 or V_2.

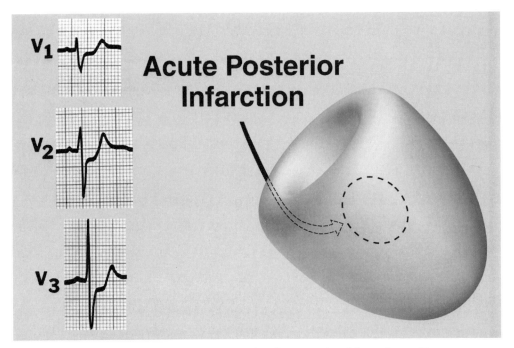

In summary, acute posterior infarction is characterized by a large R wave and ST depression in V_1 or V_2 (sometimes even in V_3).

NOTE: Always be suspicious of ST segment depression in the right chest leads, for it could indicate an acute posterior infarction. If you do not remember those things that can cause ST depression, look back at page 255. The diagnosis (page 256) of an "anterior subendocardial infarction" (because of depressed ST segments in chest leads) should be made only with extreme caution, because this ST depression may actually represent an acute true posterior infarct.

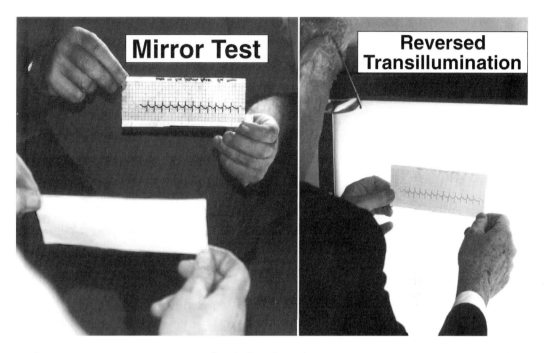

If you suspect an acute posterior infarction (large R wave and ST depression in V_1 or V_2), then try "reversed trans-illumination" or the "mirror test."

NOTE: If acute posterior infarction is suspected because of tall R waves and ST depression in V_1 or V_2 — try *reversed trans-illumination* or the *mirror test.* Both of these tests require that you invert the tracing first.

- Reversed trans-illumination: First, *invert the EKG tracing*, then hold the inverted tracing so that it faces a strong light. Observe the back side of the tracing to check for "Q waves and ST depression" in the inverted V_1 and V_2 leads.   ) elevation ?

- Mirror Test: First, *invert the EKG tracing*, then observe it in a mirror. If there is an acute posterior infarction, you will see the classic signs of "Q waves and ST elevation" in the reflection of the inverted V_1 and V_2 leads.

NOTE: With either test, remember to first *invert the tracing*. Then face the tracing toward a mirror for the mirror test; or for reversed trans-illumination, place the tracing in front of a strong light, viewing the EKG through its back side.

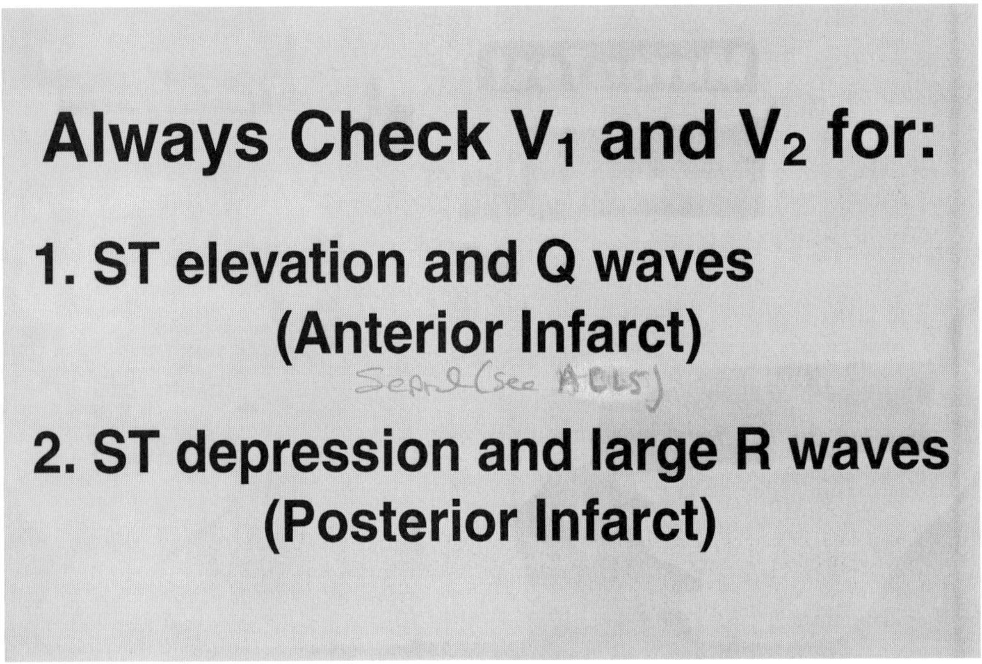

Always Check V₁ and V₂ for:

1. ST elevation and Q waves (Anterior Infarct)

Sept 2 (see ACLS)

2. ST depression and large R waves (Posterior Infarct)

Although posterior infarctions are severe, they are easy to overlook.

When making your routine reading of an EKG, pay special attention to leads V_1 and ___ while looking for signs of infarction.

V_2

NOTE: ST changes in V_1 and V_2 are always significant and important...both depression AND elevation.

Check for Q waves in V_1 and V_2 and be sure to observe the height of the __ waves.

R

NOTE: And remember how important T wave inversion can be in all leads.

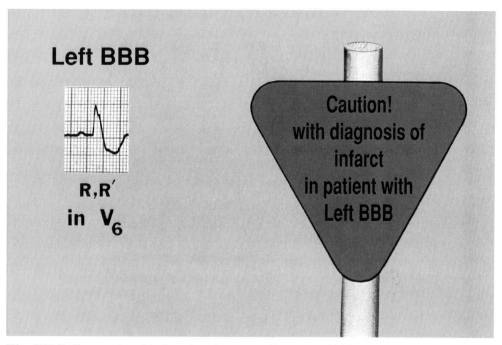

Left BBB

R,R′

in V₆

Caution!
with diagnosis of
infarct
in patient with
Left BBB

The EKG diagnosis of infarction is generally not valid in the presence of Left Bundle Branch Block.

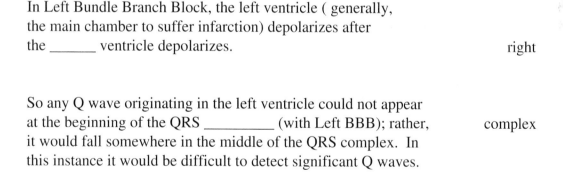

In Left Bundle Branch Block, the left ventricle (generally, the main chamber to suffer infarction) depolarizes after the _____ ventricle depolarizes.

right

So any Q wave originating in the left ventricle could not appear at the beginning of the QRS _____ (with Left BBB); rather, it would fall somewhere in the middle of the QRS complex. In this instance it would be difficult to detect significant Q waves.

complex

NOTE: One special exception is possible. The right and left ventricles share the interventricular septum in common. So an infarct in the septal area would be shared by the right ventricle, which depolarizes first in Left BBB. This would produce Q waves at the beginning of the wide QRS. Therefore, even in the presence of Left BBB, Q waves in the chest leads might suggest (but not confirm) septal (anterior) infarction.

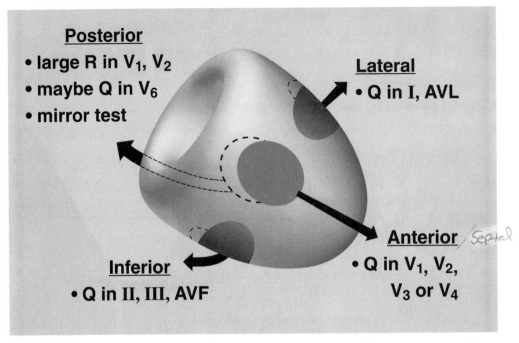

Posterior
- **large R in V_1, V_2**
- **maybe Q in V_6**
- **mirror test**

Lateral
- **Q in I, AVL**

Anterior Septal
- **Q in V_1, V_2, V_3 or V_4**

Inferior
- **Q in II, III, AVF**

Locating an infarct is important because treatment modalities and prognosis depend on the location of the infarction.

There are four general locations within the _____ ventricle   left
where infarctions commonly occur.

NOTE: More than one area of the left ventricle may infarct. One infarction
may be very old, while another is very recent (acute). So correlate the
ST elevation with the appropriate leads both to locate, and to determine the
acuteness of each infarct. If ST elevation is present in leads *without* Q waves,
"non-Q wave infarction" must be ruled out.

Be careful about diagnosing an infarction in the presence of _____   Left
Bundle Branch Block.

NOTE: Isolated areas of Ischemia (T wave inversion) or ST elevation
without Q's (for non-Q wave infarction) can also be "located" by
using the same location criteria.

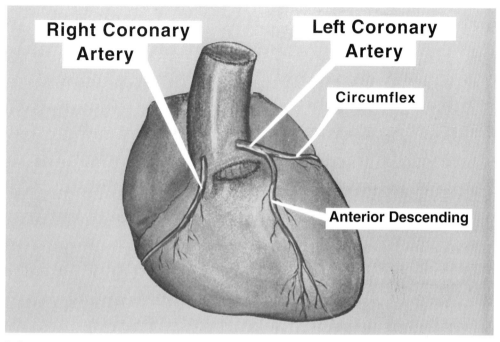

It is common practice to determine the location of an infarction, but with a little anatomical knowledge of the heart's coronary blood supply*, we can make a far more sophisticated diagnosis.

There are two coronary arteries that provide the heart with a continuous supply of oxygenated _____.   blood

Quickly review the illustration.
The *Left Coronary Artery* has two major branches; they are the *Circumflex* branch and the _____ *Descending* branch.   *Anterior*

The *Right Coronary Artery* curves around the right

_____.   ventricle

* The pulmonary artery has been "surgically" removed in this illustration to show the origin of the coronary arteries at the base of the aorta.

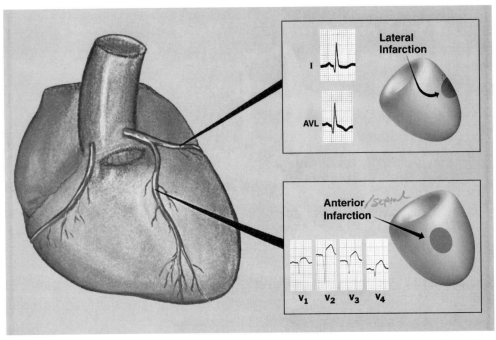

A *lateral infarction* is caused by an occlusion of the Circumflex branch of the Left Coronary Artery. An anterior infarction is due to an occlusion of the Anterior Descending branch of the Left Coronary Artery.

The Circumflex branch of the Left Coronary Artery distributes blood to the _____ portion of the left ventricle.

lateral

The Anterior Descending branch of the Left Coronary Artery supplies blood to the anterior portion of the _____ ventricle.

left

The Circumflex and the Anterior Descending are the two main branches of the _____ Coronary Artery.

Left

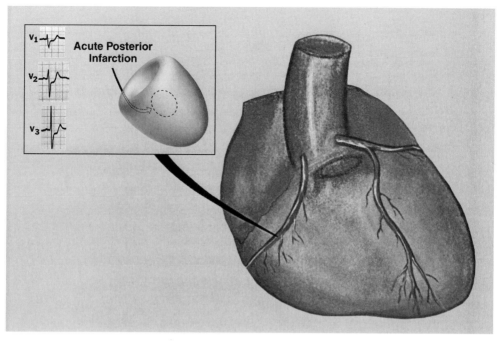

True posterior infarctions are generally caused by an occlusion of the Right Coronary Artery or one of its branches. *Like Posterior descending*

The Right Coronary Artery wraps around the right ventricle posteriorly to supply the _____ portion of the left ventricle.   posterior

So a posterior infarction usually is caused by an occlusion of a branch of the _____ Coronary Artery.   Right

NOTE: For a long time the Right Coronary Artery was thought to play only a minor role in supplying blood to the heart. Sophisticated techniques of cardiac catheterization and coronary angiography have shown that the Right Coronary Artery usually provides the blood supply to the SA Node, the AV Node, and the His Bundle. It is no wonder that acute posterior infarction is often associated with serious arrhythmias. Wise health care providers treat posterior infarction with concern and respect.

Arlys Book says His Bundle - lad - septal Branch.
Another Source has his done By RCA.

275

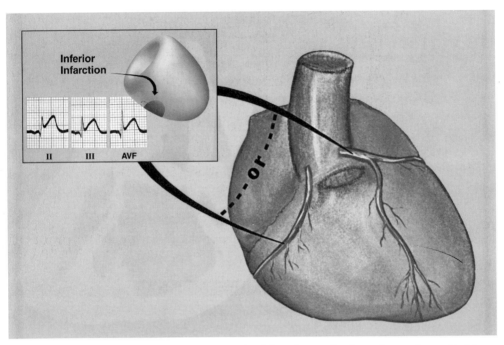

The base of the left ventricle receives its blood supply from branches of either the Right or the Left Coronary Artery, depending on which artery is "dominant."

Inferior ("diaphragmatic") infarctions are caused by an occluded terminal branch of either the Right or the _____ Coronary Artery.

Left

So the diagnosis of inferior infarction does not necessarily identify the artery branch that is occluded, unless you have a previous coronary arteriogram (an x-ray highlighting the coronary arteries) to identify which _____ artery supplies the inferior portion of that patient's left ventricle.

coronary

NOTE: Left or Right Coronary "dominance" denotes which coronary artery is the major source of blood supply to the base of the left ventricle. Right Coronary dominance is by far most common in humans.

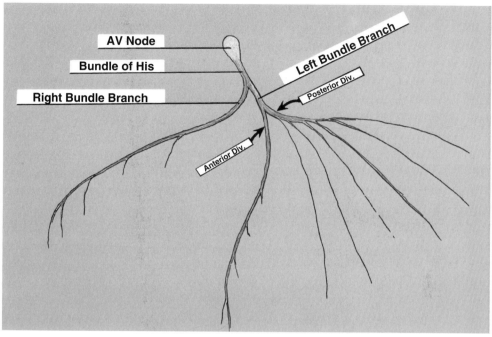

Hemiblocks are presented in this section (Infarction) because they commonly occur with infarction and an associated diminished blood supply to one of the two divisions of the Left Bundle Branch.

NOTE: The Left Bundle Branch subdivides into two divisions.

The hemiblocks are blocks of either the Anterior or the Posterior Division of the _____ Bundle Branch.   Left

Hemiblocks are commonly due to loss of blood supply to either the Anterior or the Posterior _____ of the Left   Division
Bundle Branch.

NOTE: The Right Bundle Branch does not have consistent, named subdivisions of either clinical or electrocardiographic importance (yet).

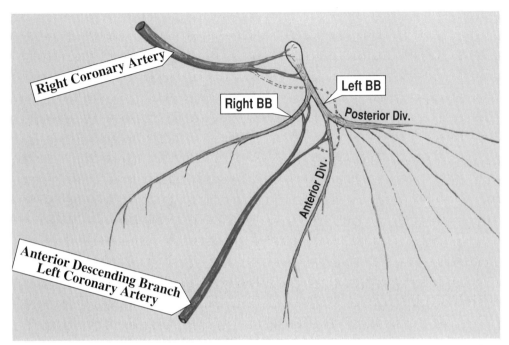

To understand hemiblocks, you must know the blood supply to the AV Node and the ventricular conduction system. Follow text and illustration closely.

The Right Coronary Artery usually renders a blood supply*
to the AV Node, Bundle of His and a variable twig to the
Posterior Division of the Left _____ Branch.   Bundle

The Left Coronary Artery also sends a variable twig to
the Posterior Division of the Left Bundle _____.   Branch

A total occlusion of the Anterior Descending branch of the
Left Coronary Artery may cause a subsequent Right Bundle Branch
_____ with an Anterior Hemiblock (a block of the Anterior   Block
Division of the Left Bundle Branch). Study the illustration carefully.

NOTE: The key to knowing hemiblocks is understanding that an infarction
may be due to an occlusion of a vessel at any of numerous locations, and
therefore may cause a variety of blocks of the Bundle Branch system.
There can be single blocks of a bundle or division, or combinations of these
blocks, that spare one or more branches. A coronary obstruction that is
not quite complete may cause an *intermittent* block.

* Let's not forget that the SA Node is usually dependent on the right coronary artery.

278

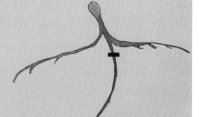

Anterior Hemiblock

- **L.A.D. - usually assoc. with an M.I. (or other heart disease)**

- **QRS slightly widened (.10 to .12)**

- **$Q_1 S_3$**

Anterior Hemiblock refers to a block of the Anterior Division of the Left Bundle Branch, and the above criteria are used in the diagnosis.

The slight delay of conduction to the antero-lateral and superior area of the left ventricle causes (late) unopposed depolarization upward and leftward, recognized on EKG as Left _____ Deviation. Acute LAD is usually what makes you suspect Anterior Hemiblock.

Axis

With pure Anterior Hemiblock, the QRS is widened only .10 to .12 sec., but association with other blocks of the Bundle _____ system may widen the QRS more.

Branch

Anterior Hemiblock is a block of the Anterior Division of the Left Bundle Branch. Finding a Q in I and a wide and/or deep ___ in III ("$Q_1 S_3$") helps to confirm the diagnosis of Anterior Hemiblock.

S

NOTE: Previous EKG's are essential in making Anterior (or any) Hemiblock diagnosis. You *must* always rule out pre-existing sources of Left Axis Deviation, e.g., Left Ventricular Hypertrophy, "horizontal heart," or Inferior Infarction.

Anterior Hemiblock

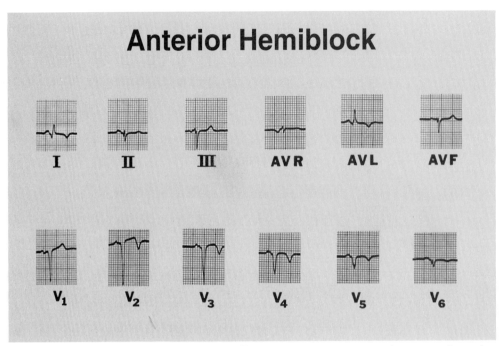

An occlusion of the Anterior Descending coronary artery produces an Anterior Infarction, and about one-half of these patients develop Anterior Hemiblock. Study the illustration on page 278.

Anterior Hemiblock is a block of the Anterior Division
of the Left Bundle Branch, which produces unopposed, late
superior-leftward depolarization in the left ventricle,
resulting in Left Axis _____.

Deviation

An occlusion of the *Anterior* Descending coronary artery
will produce an *Anterior* Infarction, which often causes
Anterior _____. (That's easy to remember.)

Hemiblock

If a patient with an acute Anterior Infarction has an associated
Axis change from normal to -60°, you should suspect
Anterior _____ (and look for Q_1S_3).

Hemiblock

But if a patient with an Inferior Infarction develops Left Axis
Deviation, don't jump to hasty conclusions! Inferior Infarction
can cause LAD, so _____ Hemiblock may not be the
culprit.

Anterior

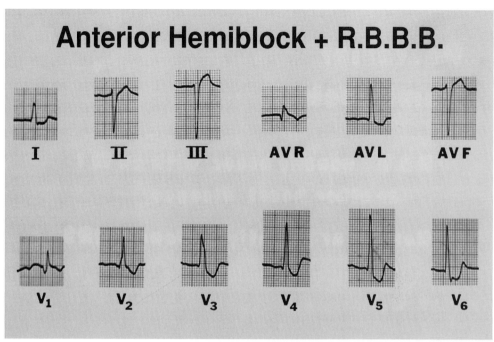

Anterior Hemiblock + R.B.B.B.

An infarction of the anterior wall of the left ventricle (due to an occluded Anterior Descending branch of the Left Coronary Artery) may cause Anterior Hemiblock <u>and</u> Right Bundle Branch Block. Review the illustration on page 278.

NOTE: Don't forget that the Anterior Descending also renders blood supply to the Right Bundle Branch, so Anterior Infarction may have an associated Right Bundle Branch Block, depending on the location of occlusion.

With Right Bundle Branch Block, the Mean QRS Vector is within the normal range or shows minimal Right Axis _____.   Deviation

However, when a patient develops a Right Bundle Branch Block with Left Axis Deviation as well, this is probably caused by Anterior Hemiblock, particularly if there is an acute Anterior _____.   Infarction

Posterior Hemiblock

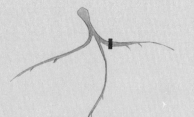

- **R.A.D.** - usually assoc. with an M.I. (or other heart disease)

- **Normal or slightly widened QRS**

- S_1Q_3

Pure, isolated *Posterior Hemiblock* is rare because the posterior division is short, thick, and commonly has a dual blood supply. See the illustration on page 278.

An inferior infarction may impair the blood supply to the Posterior division of the Left Bundle _____.

Branch

Posterior Hemiblocks cause Right Axis _____ due to the late, unopposed depolarization forces toward the right.

Deviation

When Posterior Hemiblock is suspected, look for a deep or unusually wide S in I and Q in III (known as S_1Q_3) to help confirm the _____ of Posterior Hemiblock.

diagnosis

Posterior Hemiblock

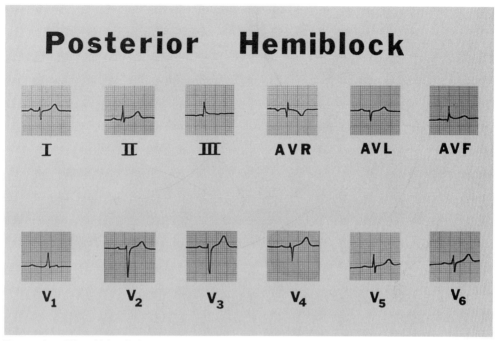

Posterior Hemiblock is always to be respected, and all Inferior Infarctions should be scrutinized to rule it out.

A lateral infarction, either recent or old, can cause Right Axis Deviation, which can be confused with Posterior Hemiblock. In the presence of a _____ M.I., the EKG diagnosis of Posterior Hemiblock is equivocal.

lateral

Make certain that by history and previous EKG's, chronic Right Axis Deviation due to slender body build ("vertical heart"), _____ Ventricular Hypertrophy, and pulmonary disease, etc. are ruled out.

Right

NOTE: Posterior Hemiblock is serious, and when associated with Right Bundle Branch Block, this combination is considered very dangerous because of the tendency to progress into AV Blocks.

IMPORTANT !: AV Block refers to "atrio-ventricular block", that is, a block between atrial depolarization and ventricular depolarization, so we commonly think of a block in the AV Node or in the His Bundle. However, simultaneous blocks of both Bundle Branches can block AV conduction. Also, RBBB in association with the simultaneous blocks of *both* divisions of the Left Bundle Branch can produce a block of AV conduction. Please contemplate that for a while.

Bifascicular Blocks

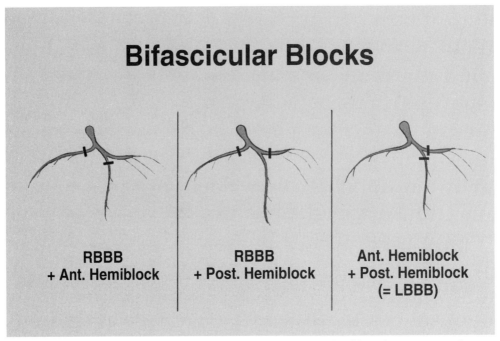

| RBBB
+ Ant. Hemiblock | RBBB
+ Post. Hemiblock | Ant. Hemiblock
+ Post. Hemiblock
(= LBBB) |

The word "fascicle" means bundle (bundle of Purkinje fibers), so any main division of the ventricular conduction system is a fascicle. This includes both Bundle Branches as well as both Divisions of the Left Bundle Branch.

NOTE: Previously, "Bundle" implied only the Right or the Left Bundle Branch. But now, to avoid confusion, combinations of blocks (e.g., Hemiblock + Bundle Branch Block) we use a more inclusive term, "fascicular" block, to denote a Bundle Branch Block with a Hemiblock.

NOTE: "Bifascicular" block means that two fascicles are blocked. Anterior Hemiblock plus Posterior Hemiblock is clinically the same as Left Bundle Branch Block. So Bifascicular Block generally refers to Right Bundle Branch Block together with a block of either the Anterior Division or the Posterior Division (of the Left Bundle Branch).

NOTE: A block of both the Right and the Left Bundle Branch is a Complete AV Block. Right BBB plus a block of both the Anterior and Posterior Divisions (of the Left Bundle Branch) is also a Complete AV Block. Complete AV Block is very serious since only a ventricular focus remains to *s l o w l y* pace the ventricles...so slowly that syncope often occurs (airway!), and human life is at stake.

NOTE: When Bundle Branch Blocks or fascicular blocks are *intermittent*, we don't see them continuously on monitor or EKG tracing; just occasionally.

Intermittent Block

Intermittent block of one fascicle:
continuous EKG pattern of normal –
- with intermittent wide QRS pattern characteristic of the type of *intermittent* BBB present.
- or with intermittent change of QRS Axis (i.e. QRS orientation changes intermittently) typical of the type of *intermittent* hemiblock present.

Intermittent block of two fascicles:
- intermittent change of Axis (i.e. QRS orientation changes intermittently) characteristic of the type of *intermittent* hemiblock present.
- or intermittent wide QRS pattern characteristic of the type of *intermittent* BBB present.

Permanent block + Intermittent block:
- continuous EKG signs of one permanent block with *intermittent* EKG signs of another block.

Fortunately, combinations of (fascicular) blocks are often *intermittent*, making them quite obvious. Intermittent change in QRS axis (e.g., upright QRS's that transiently change to downward QRS's) usually indicates *intermittent* hemiblock, and a steady rhythm with transiently widened QRS's suggests *intermittent* BBB.

Intermittent block may exist in more than one fascicle in the same patient, producing a variety of transient changes of _____ Axis   QRS (intermittent [anterior or posterior] hemiblock) or...

transiently widened QRS's typical of intermittent (left or right) _____   BBB on EKG or cardiac monitor*. Don't ignore these intermittent changes; document them and give proper notification.

NOTE: Like a failing light bulb that occasionally flickers or goes off, sick fascicles may suffer intermittent block. As a failing, flickering light bulb eventually burns out, similarly, intermittent fascicular blocks often warn of impending permanent block of the fascicle. With a pre-existing permanent block of another fascicle, intermittent fascicular block can be a timely warning (the only warning!) of an imminent complete block (that's why the first word on this page is "fortunately"). In most cases, permanent block plus intermittent block is an indication for an artificial pacemaker.

*It is important and challenging to differentiate between [intermittent] anterior and posterior hemiblock, as well as [intermittent] right and left Bundle Branch Block. You know how already, but a little review wouldn't hurt.

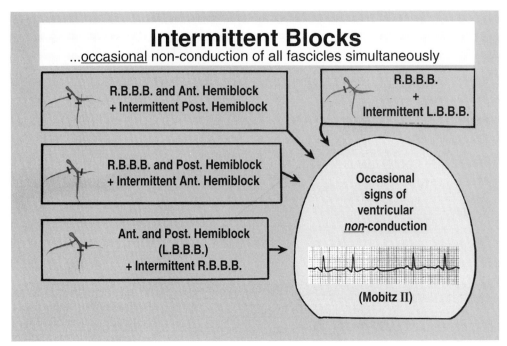

Intermittent Blocks
...occasional non-conduction of all fascicles simultaneously

| R.B.B.B. and Ant. Hemiblock + Intermittent Post. Hemiblock | R.B.B.B. + Intermittent L.B.B.B. |

R.B.B.B. and Post. Hemiblock + Intermittent Ant. Hemiblock

Ant. and Post. Hemiblock (L.B.B.B.) + Intermittent R.B.B.B.

Occasional signs of ventricular *non*-conduction

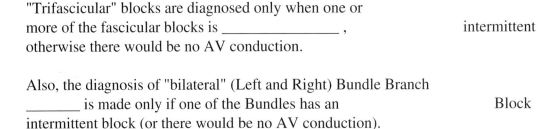

(Mobitz II)

Considering the three pathways of ventricular depolarization, it becomes apparent that one fascicle must remain functional at least intermittently to provide AV conduction. Early detection allows for early intervention.

"Trifascicular" blocks are diagnosed only when one or more of the fascicular blocks is _____ ,   intermittent
otherwise there would be no AV conduction.

Also, the diagnosis of "bilateral" (Left and Right) Bundle Branch
_____ is made only if one of the Bundles has an   Block
intermittent block (or there would be no AV conduction).

NOTE: If all fascicles are permanently blocked except one that has an intermittent block, then an intermittent Mobitz II pattern (occasional non-conduction to the ventricles) will emerge. If that Mobitz II pattern becomes more frequent in the tracing, or if a continuous Mobitz 2:1 pattern begins, or worse yet, if there is a continuous high ratio Mobitz II block, there is a strong likelihood that complete AV Block is imminent and an implantable pacemaker is needed. Knowledge plus vigilance saves lives.

WARNING! With Mobitz II, every cycle missing its QRS has a regular, punctual P wave — but NEVER a premature P' wave (see NOTE, page 124). This distinction is critical!!

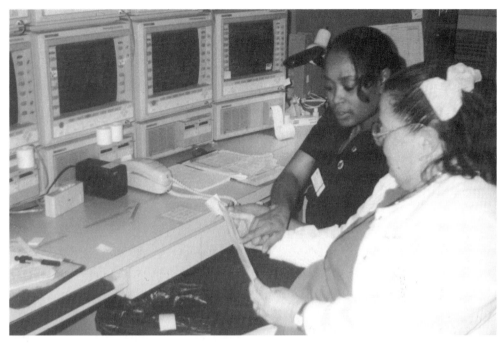

Patients with acute myocardial infarctions are placed in coronary care units and monitored continuously. In most hospitals patients with symptoms (only) of myocardial infarction receive the same cautious care. Patients with no physical symptoms of infarction but with definite EKG criteria of acute infarction ("silent infarction") require admission and monitoring also.

NOTE: Just as medical treatment of arrhythmias changes with the times, so do the attitudes toward the indications for artificial pacemakers, angioplasty with stenting, coronary bypass procedures, and thrombolytic treatment, Keep up with the changing standards in your local medical community, read the current literature, and *always know the basics.*

You should always know how to determine the location of an infarction and the vessel(s) involved, as well as their association with _____.   Hemiblocks

In patients with myocardial infarction, be alert for subtle changes of Axis (change of QRS orientation in the same lead), and also rhythm changes that may be indicative of impending _____ AV Block. Vigilance is critical.   Complete

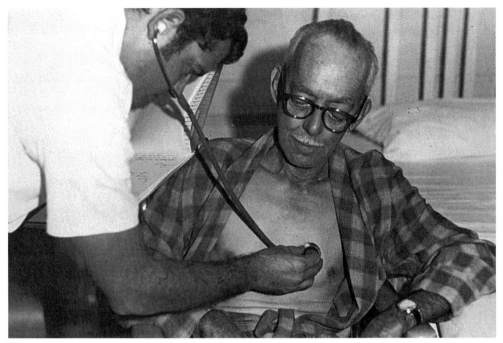

Remember that the patient's history and clinical diagnosis are still the most valuable tools you have (using your knowledge and judgment) in the determination of infarction and infarction-related problems.

The EKG has never become obsolete because it provides more
_____ information than any other diagnostic modality.   cardiac

There is no substitute for obtaining an accurate _____,   history
even if it is volunteered by witnesses to an event.

Although the laboratory provides much useful information,
the ____ is an immediate diagnostic gift for those skilled   EKG
in its interpretation.

NOTE: The value of an EKG increases multifold when it is compared to a patient's previous tracings — get them as soon as possible! Incidentally, is this a photo of Dr. Paul Dudley White, and who is his examining physician?

NOTE: Review Infarction by turning to the **P**ersonal **Q**uick **R**eference **S**heets on pages 318 to 319, and again, look at your simplified methodology (page 310).

Miscellaneous Effects

Pulmonary

Electrolytes

Medications

Artificial Pacemakers

Heart Transplants

The above effects are common to, but not necessarily diagnostic of, certain conditions or situations that can produce recognizable changes on the EKG.

NOTE: Certain effects may be recognized by their characteristic appearance on the electrocardiogram or on cardiac monitor. For most of the conditions to be discussed in this section, the electrocardiographic signs merely alert us to be aware of existing conditions, certain pathology, or drug or electrolyte effects. But to confirm your suspicion, you should review the medical history, carry out a detailed physical exam, and obtain proper diagnostic tests. Rarely is a diagnosis based entirely on any of the following EKG findings, however they are exceptionally helpful.

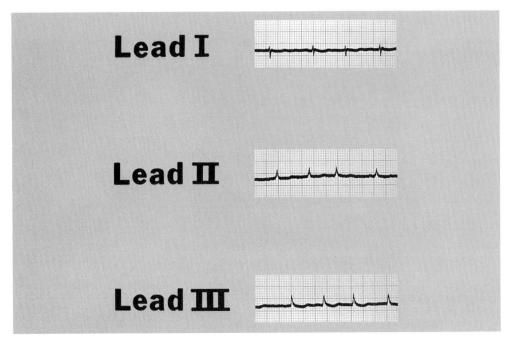

Chronic Obstructive Pulmonary Disease (COPD) often produces low voltage deflections in all leads, and there is usually Right Axis Deviation.

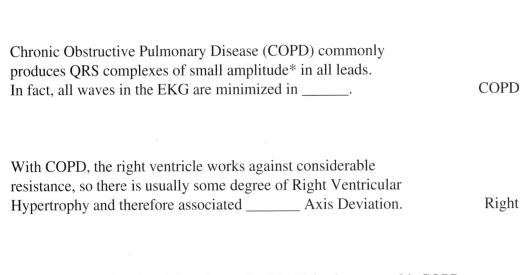

Chronic Obstructive Pulmonary Disease (COPD) commonly produces QRS complexes of small amplitude* in all leads. In fact, all waves in the EKG are minimized in _____.

COPD

With COPD, the right ventricle works against considerable resistance, so there is usually some degree of Right Ventricular Hypertrophy and therefore associated _____ Axis Deviation.

Right

NOTE: Multifocal Atrial Tachycardia (MAT) is also seen with COPD.

*Low voltage in all leads also appears with hypothyroidism and chronic constrictive pericarditis.

Pulmonary Embolus

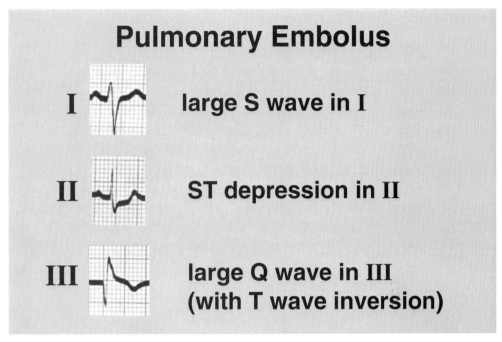

I   large S wave in I

II   ST depression in II

III   large Q wave in III
(with T wave inversion)

With *Pulmonary Embolus* we usually see a large S wave in lead I, and a Q wave and an inverted T wave in lead III ($S_1Q_3L_3$)*.

$S_1Q_3L_3$ syndrome characterizes acute *cor pulmonale* resulting from pulmonary embolus. It is called $S_1Q_3L_3$ because of the large S wave in lead I, and there is a Q wave and an inverted T wave in lead ___.   III

NOTE: Notice the typical tendency toward right Axis Deviation (lead I).

There is usually ST segment _____ in lead II.   depression

* Don't be confused by the inversion of the T in the printed text. It's a great memory tool, even if the publisher dislikes it.

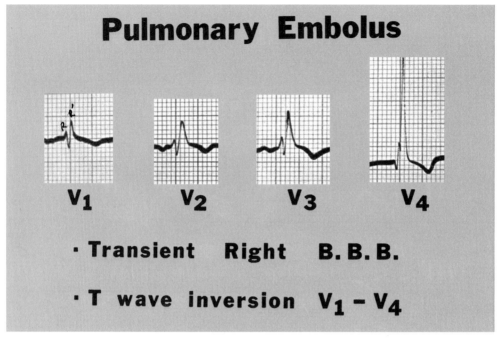

Also with pulmonary embolus, there is usually T wave inversion in V_1 through V_4. Often there is Right Bundle Branch Block.

T wave inversion in the chest leads (particularly in
leads V_1 through V_4) is a very important diagnostic
sign of pulmonary _____.   embolus

Pulmonary embolus may cause _____ Bundle Branch Block.   Right
This block often subsides after the patient improves.

We can recognize the presence of Right Bundle Branch Block
by the R,R' in the right _____ leads.   chest

NOTE: Occasionally the Right Bundle Branch Block may be "incomplete"
(QRS of normal width, but R,R' is present).

Potassium
Hyper K$^+$

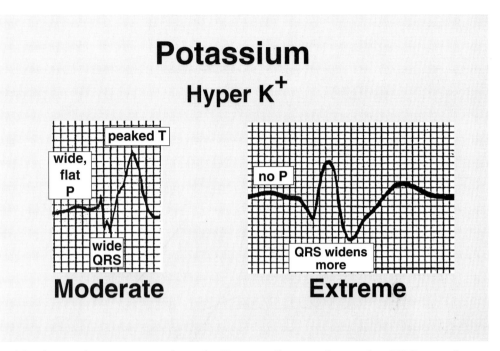

Moderate   **Extreme**

With elevated serum potassium the P wave flattens down, the QRS complex widens, and the T wave becomes peaked.

NOTE: The potassium ion (K$^+$) plays an extremely important role in cardiac electrophysiology, The range of normal serum K$^+$ concentration is very narrow. In medical parlance we add the suffix "-emia" to the end of the ion name to denote its presence in the blood...but it sounds funny with potassium. So its chemical symbol, K, is pronounced verbally, and the prefix "hyper" for increased, or the prefix "hypo" for decreased, is added to communicate deviations from normal. Now you'll understand both *hyper*- and *hypo*- kalemia* (pronounced "kay-LEE-mia"). And that's right, it's written "kalemia ." That should help you and also your friends who might be perplexed...

The most striking and classic feature of elevated serum potassium is the _____ T wave.   peaked

The P wave widens and flattens with increased serum potassium, and with extreme hyperkalemia the __ wave nearly disappears.   P

When a patient has hyperkalemia, ventricular depolarization takes longer, so the QRS complex _____.   widens

* The "l" is added to enhance the phonics, so you don't have to get the "l" out of there (chuckle!).

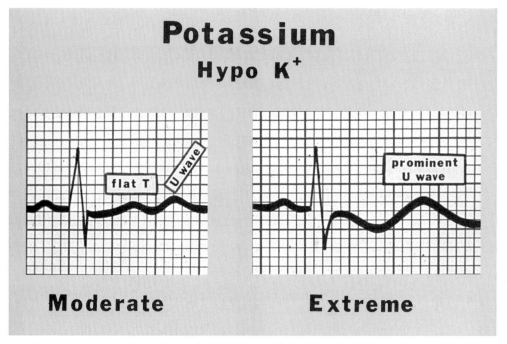

Potassium
Hypo K$^+$

flat T · U wave · **Moderate**

prominent U wave · **Extreme**

As the serum potassium drops below normal levels, the T wave becomes flat (or inverted) and a U wave appears.

With hypokalemia, as the serum potassium concentration drops, the __ wave flattens out, and if the K$^+$ concentration drops lower, the T wave inverts.

    T

NOTE: I always think of the T wave as tent housing potassium ions. When there is an increase in potassium ions the tent peaks up, but lowering of potassium ions lowers the height of the tent.

With hypokalemia a __ wave appears. This wave becomes more pronounced as the loss of potassium becomes more severe.

    U

NOTE: Potassium is not just "one of those serum electrolytes". Potassium plays a critical role in repolarization and also in maintaining a precise resting potential. A decrease in potassium makes ventricular automaticity foci extremely irritable. In fact, low potassium can initiate Torsades de Pointes, and it can also evoke dangerous ventricular tachy-arrhythmias. Hypokalemia also enhances the toxic effects of digitalis excess.

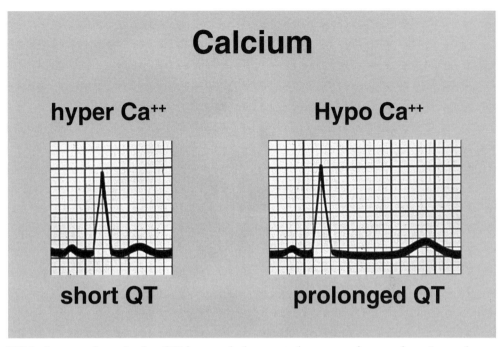

Calcium

hyper Ca⁺⁺   Hypo Ca⁺⁺

short QT   prolonged QT

With *hypercalcemia* the QT interval shortens; however *hypocalcemia* prolongs the QT interval.

NOTE: Since you already understand "hyper-" and "hypo-", I only need mention that "-calcemia" is pronounced "cal-SEE-mia".

Hypocalcemia will prolong the ___ interval.   QT

NOTE: The QT interval is measured from the beginning of the QRS complex to the end of the T wave. Normally, the QT interval should be less that half of the cycle length.

Increased serum calcium accelerates both ventricular depolarization and ventricular repolarization. This is manifested as a short
QT _____.   interval

In extreme cases of hypocalcemia there is T wave inversion.

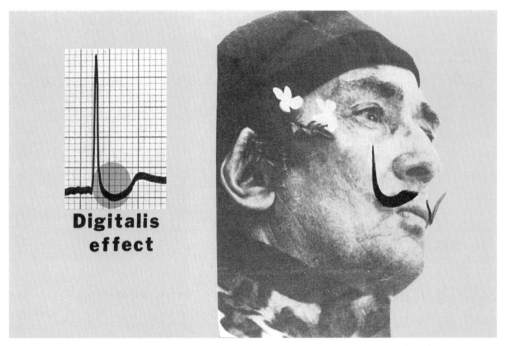

Digitalis causes a gradual down-sloping of the ST segment, to give it the appearance of Salvador Dali's mustache. Notice that the lowest portion of the ST segment is depressed below the baseline.

Digitalis produces a unique, gradual down-sloping of the
___ segment; this is the classical "digitalis effect."   ST

NOTE: To identify the classical pattern of digitalis effect, you should observe a lead with no demonstrable S wave. The downward portion of the R wave gradually thickens as it curves down into the ST segment, which is usually depressed. The downward limb of the R wave has a gentle, curving slope that gradually blends into the <u>depressed</u> ST segment. Look for it the next time you have a patient on a digitalis preparation.

NOTE: Digitalis in therapeutic doses has a parasympathetic effect. With a Sinus Rhythm, digitalis slows the rate of SA Node pacing. Conduction through the AV Node is slowed, and digitalis also inhibits the AV Node's receptiveness to multiple stimuli, allowing fewer stimuli to reach the ventricles (as with Atrial Flutter and Atrial Fibrillation) to permit a more physiological and more efficient ventricular response rate. Digitalis has a very narrow range of therapeutic effectiveness, and should this therapeutic range be exceeded, a multitude of undesirable effects can result. See the next two pages...

Excess Digitalis

- **Atrial & Junctional Premature Beats**

- **PAT with Block**

- **Sinus Block**

- **AV Blocks**

Excess digitalis tends to cause AV Blocks of many varieties, and may even induce Sinus (SA) Block.

NOTE: Supraventricular (particularly atrial) foci are exceptionally sensitive to digitalis, so PAB's are often the earliest warning sign that your patient has elevated levels of digitalis. Atrial automaticity foci are very effective digitalis sensors.

Digitalis in excess may cause transient Sinus _____.   Block

Digitalis retards conduction of depolarization through
the AV Node; and in excess, it can cause various types
of ___ Block, particularly rate-dependent AV Block.   AV

Automaticity foci of the atria and the AV Junction can
become irritable when _____ preparations are   digitalis
present in excessive concentrations in your patient.

NOTE: Low serum potassium can enhance the toxicity of digitalis,
so that digitalis, even in therapeutic concentrations, can produce undesirable
signs of toxicity if the serum potassium is low.

297

Digitalis Toxicity

- **Atrial & Junctional Tachy-arrhythmias**

- **PVC's**

- **Ventricular Bigeminy, Trigeminy**

- **Ventricular Tachycardia**

- **Ventricular Fibrillation**

Atrial and Junctional automaticity foci are very likely to become irritable in the presence of excessive digitalis. In fact, marked *digitalis toxicity* can even provoke ventricular foci into rapid and dangerous rhythms.

The foci of the atria and AV Junction are most sensitive to excessive digitalis, but with marked digitalis _____, even ventricular foci may become so irritable that they may spontaneously emit PVC's.

toxicity

Marked digitalis toxicity can make ventricular foci so irritable that they may suddenly fire multiple discharges that initiate dangerous _____ tachy-arrhythmias.

ventricular

NOTE: Digitalis preparations have been used medicinally by civilized people since the thirteenth century. But like most other cardiac medications, in certain circumstances or in high concentrations deadly arrhythmias may arise.

Quinidine Effects

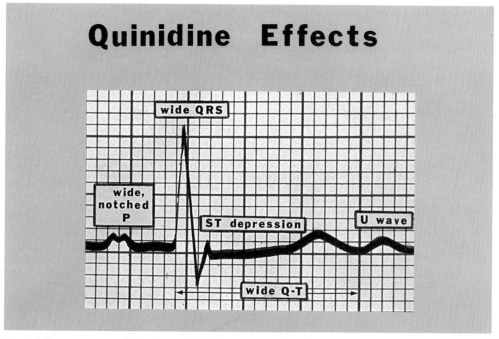

Quinidine causes widening of the P wave and widening of the QRS complex. There is often ST depression with a prolonged QT. The presence of U waves is typical as well.

NOTE: Quinidine retards depolarization and repolarization through both the atrial and the ventricular myocardium. Most of the effects of quinidine that we see on EKG relate to its pharmacological effects on sodium and potassium channel blockade.

Quinidine causes a wide, notched ___ wave on EKG, and the QRS complex is also widened.   P

Quinidine prolongs the ___ interval, and depresses the ST segment. Look for U waves (which represent delayed repolarization of the ventricular conduction system).   QT

NOTE: Episodes of Torsades de Pointes - a rapid and dangerous ventricular rhythm can result from quinidine toxicity (see page 153).

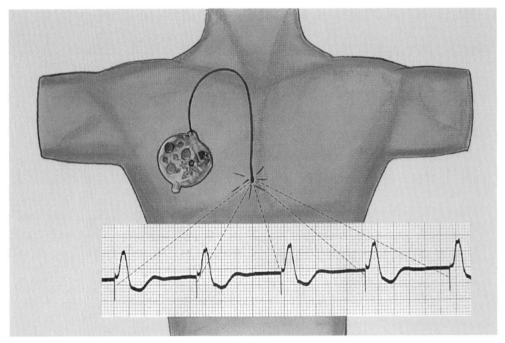

Artificial pacemakers have a pulse generator with a long-lasting battery.
The pacemaking stimuli are designed for ventricular or atrial (or both)
pacing modalities, and a wide variety of sensing features are available.

NOTE Artificial pacemakers are surgically implanted as a permanent
pacemaking source. Originally, they were designed to counter the
bradycardia that attends Complete AV Block and Sick Sinus Syndrome.
Now, the uses and variety of pacemaker types is well beyond the scope of
this book, so we will review only basic principles of artificial cardiac pacing.
In most cases the pacemaker electrode leads are passed transvenously into
the right side of the heart; however, sometimes the stimulating electrodes
are surgically attached to the epicardial surface of the heart.

The pacemaker generator emits regular pacing stimuli, which
record on the _____ as a narrow vertical spike.   EKG

The pacemaker emits regular paced electrical _____,   stimuli
and each stimulus should "capture" (i.e., depolarize) the myocardial
tissue in contact with the electrode. The depolarization stimulus
then conducts through the myocardium.

300

Demand Pacemaker

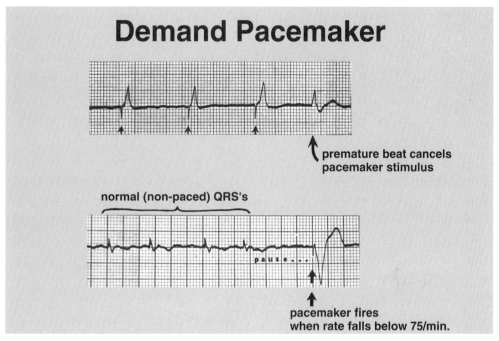

premature beat cancels
pacemaker stimulus

normal (non-paced) QRS's

pause....

pacemaker fires
when rate falls below 75/min.

The *Demand* feature of many artificial pacemakers is designed to imitate the physiological mechanisms of an automaticity focus (great idea!). The Demand pacemaker is programmed with an "inherent rate" that is overdrive-suppressed by normal Sinus pacing.

NOTE: The illustration depicts a Demand pacemaker with a ventricular sensing electrode and a ventricular pacing electrode.

A Demand pacemaker is *overdrive-suppressed* by normal Sinus pacing, but should the Sinus rate drop below the pacemaker's programmed inherent rate, the pacemaker, no longer overdrive-suppressed, escapes to assume pacemaking responsibility at its inherent _____.   rate

But if the SA Node resumes pacing at a normal rate (which is faster than the _____ rate of the Demand pacemaker) the   inherent
Demand pacemaker is overdrive-suppressed and stops pacing.

The Demand pacemaker is designed to *reset* just like an automaticity focus. When the Demand pacemaker senses a PVC, it resets its pacing (at the cycle length of its inherent rate) in step with the ____ .   PVC
This provides for uninterrupted cardiac function (clever engineers design to imitate Nature).

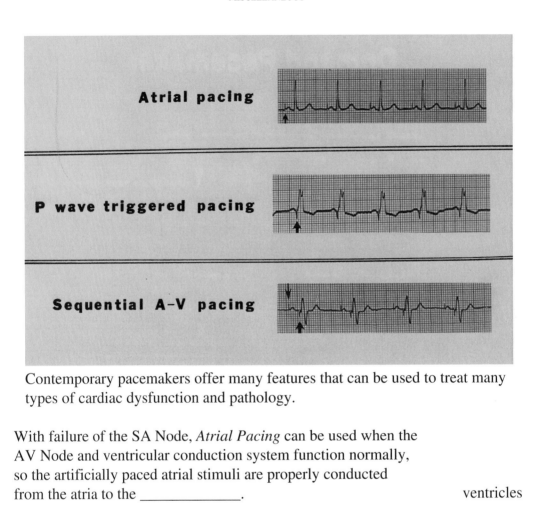

Atrial pacing

P wave triggered pacing

Sequential A-V pacing

Contemporary pacemakers offer many features that can be used to treat many types of cardiac dysfunction and pathology.

With failure of the SA Node, *Atrial Pacing* can be used when the AV Node and ventricular conduction system function normally, so the artificially paced atrial stimuli are properly conducted from the atria to the _____.

ventricles

A Complete AV Block may prevent normal Sinus pacing from conducting to the ventricles and may require *P wave triggered pacing*, which senses the __ wave, then after a brief pause (imitating normal AV conduction) it generates a stimulus for ventricular depolarization.

P

SA Node malfunction combined with Complete AV Block sometimes necessitates *Sequential AV pacing,* which provides a stimulus for atrial depolarization followed by a brief pause, then the ventricles are _____.

depolarized

NOTE: Modern pacemakers are computerized wonders that can detect and respond to physiological needs such as decreased rate during sleep and increased rate during exercise.

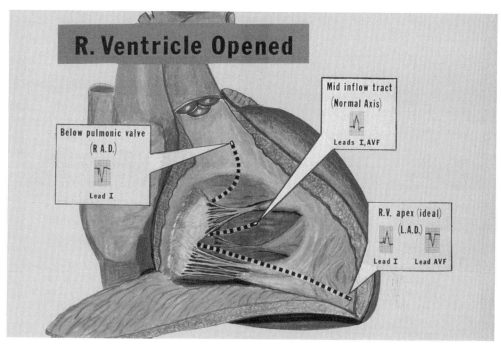

Usually a right ventricular electrode is used for cardiac pacemaking; the electrode tip of the lead is positioned within the cavity of the right ventricle. Three catheter lead positions are shown with the way they record on EKG.

NOTE: For the ideal placement of a right ventricular pacemaker lead, the electrode tip is permanently placed in the apex of the right ventricle. The resultant QRS complex has a Left Bundle Branch Block pattern with Left Axis Deviation.

When a paced QRS shows a LBBB _____ with a normal axis, the electrode tip is in the mid-inflow tract of the right ventricle.

pattern

But if you notice a paced QRS with a LBBB pattern and Right Axis Deviation, the tip of the _____ is just below the pulmonic valves.

electrode

NOTE: Certain cardiac patients may have a surgically implanted "pacemaker", called an *Implantable Cardioverter Defibrillator* (ICD) that can pace, detect and interpret rhythm disturbances, and treat tachyarrhythmias by overdrive pacing or cardioversion, even defibrillate in the event of ventricular fibrillation. Oh, Brave New World!

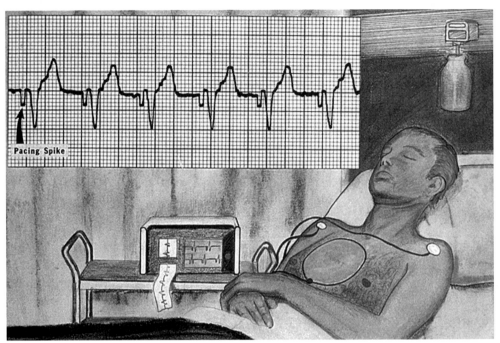

There is an *external non-invasive* pacemaking device that effectively delivers pacing stimuli to the heart through intact skin in emergency situations.

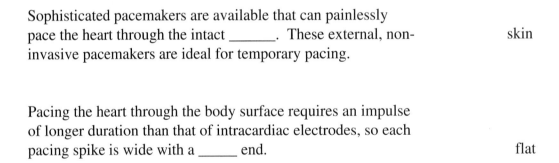

Sophisticated pacemakers are available that can painlessly pace the heart through the intact _____. These external, non-invasive pacemakers are ideal for temporary pacing.

skin

Pacing the heart through the body surface requires an impulse of longer duration than that of intracardiac electrodes, so each pacing spike is wide with a _____ end.

flat

NOTE: Another externally applied emergency device, the *Automated External Defibrillator* (AED), records and analyses the patient's EKG, and then automatically defibrillates the patient if a deadly arrhythmia is detected. The AED is very accurate in its computerized recognition of Ventricular Fibrillation and high rate Ventricular Tachycardia, and it provides considerable ease of use by moderately trained personnel. Numerous trials and studies have proven the AED to be a very effective method of defibrillation in a non-hospital setting.

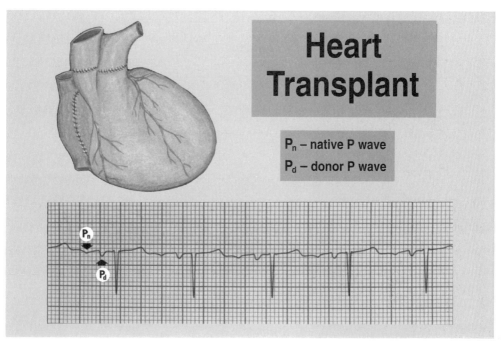

A *heart transplant* procedure leaves portions of the recipient patient's "native" atria in place. These portions of atria contain the patient's own SA Node, so the transplant patient has his native SA Node, plus the SA Node of the donor heart.

NOTE: To be expeditious during these procedures, the portions of the native atria that contain the large vessel orifices are left behind to be sutured to the atria of the transplanted heart. So the recipient patient retains his native SA Node, and the donor heart that he receives also has a functioning SA Node.

Transplant patients therefore have two SA Nodes, each producing ___ waves. P

The native SA Node produces depolarizations that do not pass beyond the suture line, so they do not depolarize the donor _____. atria

The transplanted heart has its own functional SA Node that is its dominant pacemaker, so all of its P waves are followed by ___ complexes. QRS

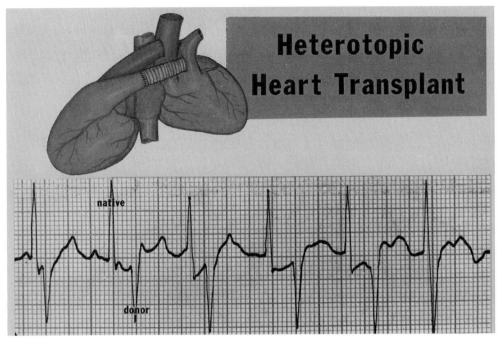

A *heterotopic* heart transplant is a procedure that leaves the native heart
in place, while a temporary, donor heart is surgically attached to assist the
pumping effort.

In order to assist in pumping a heterotopic heart transplant
gives the patient (temporarily) two _____.   hearts

So the EKG in this temporary, emergency situation displays
the simultaneous recording of the electrical activity of two
separate _____.   hearts

NOTE: With great advances in medical technology and increasing
sophistication of biomechanical engineering, attempts are constantly being
made to devise an efficient artificial heart. It is unlikely that a totally artificial
heart will ever approach the efficacy and safety of that Designed by Nature.

Let me know if your understanding was a kind of ecstacy.
(It has been for me.) –DD

Cardiac Monitor Displays

Cardiac monitors display the same information as recorded on a standard 12 lead EKG. Some initial apprehension may arise because of lack of familiarity with the display. There is an increased amplitude of waves (height and depth) as well as a reversal of customary black tracing on white EKG paper, and some monitors lack a background grid. But don't despair, this is just another method of displaying the heart's electrical activity...and familiarity eventually breeds content.

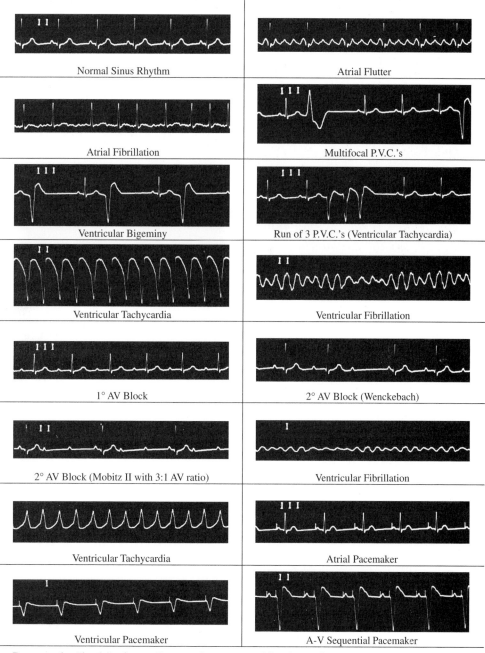

Normal Sinus Rhythm	Atrial Flutter
Atrial Fibrillation	Multifocal P.V.C.'s
Ventricular Bigeminy	Run of 3 P.V.C.'s (Ventricular Tachycardia)
Ventricular Tachycardia	Ventricular Fibrillation
1° AV Block	2° AV Block (Wenckebach)
2° AV Block (Mobitz II with 3:1 AV ratio)	Ventricular Fibrillation
Ventricular Tachycardia	Atrial Pacemaker
Ventricular Pacemaker	A-V Sequential Pacemaker

Because the "leads" of a cardiac monitor are modifications of standard leads with exaggerated amplitudes to aid in visualization at a distance, voltage (height and depth) criteria can not be utilized.

Monitor Displays Courtesy of Marquette Electronics, Inc.
Milwaukee, WI, U.S.A.

> **Electrocardiography was your challenge; knowledge, your achievement.**

Now that you are certainly pleased with your understanding of basic electrocardiography, and proud of your ability to interpret the information on EKG's and cardiac monitors, you realize how logical and marvelously Designed is the heart.

You're probably ready for *Heart,* Dr. Dubin's work in progress. For your giant leap into the 21st century, when your knowledge will need to be on a molecular level, let Dr. Dubin be your guide and simplify your understanding. Here is an edited summary of the advance pre-publication release.

*Heart is an exciting full-color expedition deep into the secret molecular wonderland of cardiac physiology with a splash of biochemistry. We will explore the vivid inner world of the magnificent "ion movers", a dynamic microcosm of exotic **ion channels**, **ion pumps**, **ion exchangers**, the mysterious **connexons,** and the fast moving ions they control. You will be immersed in this never-before-seen, living wonderland that generates the heart's electrical energy and power responding to physiological demands. What a performance to behold, as we expose the private activities of these ion movers exquisitely orchestrated by the autonomic nervous system. Heart is narrated in Dr. Dubin's entertaining, easy to understand style as you discover what really makes the healthy heart tick, yet falter with stress and disease. Though this adventure will likely not become a great movie, it is the beautiful, illustrated story of the intimate lifestyles of the ions and their movers as recorded by the surface EKG.*

*See last page, inside back cover.

COVER Publishing Company
P.O. Box 1092
Tampa, FL 33601
U. S. A.

308

Heart, a work in progress, is an exciting adventure in living color, providing vital knowledge for the medical profession in millennium 2000.

Scientists and researchers in the twentieth century found the micro-structure of the cells of the heart to be an engineering wonder. Research continues to reveal intriguing information, while raising many new questions. Current concepts may seem complex–even intimidating–to medical professionals, although, in reality, they are easy to understand.

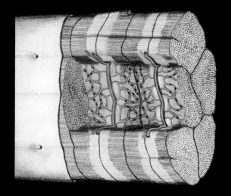

The key to cardiac function is at the ionic-molecular level, where autonomic control occurs, and where medications work. All the electrical and mechanical properties of the heart are due to the movement of only three types of ions...yes, three little ions!

Let me have them come forward to introduce them by name:

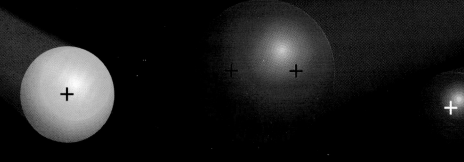

Sodium ion (Na$^+$)　　　　Calcium ion (Ca^{++})　　　Potassium ion (K$^+$)

Ion-moving ("ion-kinetic") mechanisms of the cell membrane (and cell interior) create the circumstances that cause ion movement. Most of these mechanisms are sophisticated molecular portals that control and regulate the movement of Na^+, Ca^{++}, and K^+ ions. Each variety of ion-kinetic mechanism has its own unique behavior.

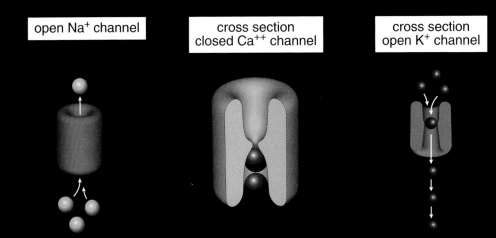

open Na^+ channel

cross section
closed Ca^{++} channel

cross section
open K^+ channel

We are launching an expedition to explore this incredible ionic-molecular microcosm to learn just how these mechanisms move Na^+, Ca^{++}, and K^+ ions to govern the heart's function. We would love to have you join us on this fascinating adventure.

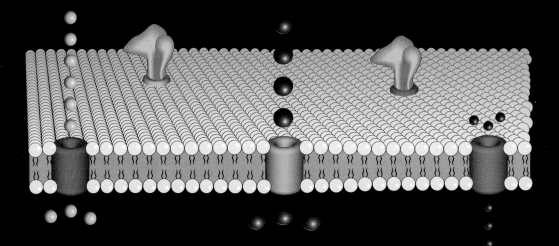

Our fantastic journey is narrated by a five year old boy named Dale, so certainly anyone who has read *Rapid Interpretation of EKG's* can easily master this vital medical knowledge, which is so useful and necessary in millennium 2000.

Hurry...your knowledge is needed!

Personal Quick Reference Sheets

(pages 309 to 322)

from: Dubin's *Rapid Interpretation of EKG's*
published by: COVER Publishing Co., P.O. Box 1092, Tampa, FL 33601, USA

The owner of this book is encouraged to copy pages 309 through 322 to carry as a personal quick reference, however, copying for or by others is strictly prohibited. The entire text of *Rapid Interpretation of EKG's* is fully protected by domestic United States copyright as well as the Universal Copyright Convention, and all rights of absolute imprimatur are enforced by COVER Publishing Co.

RAPID
INTERPRETATION
OF
EKG's

Dubin's classic, simplified methodology for understanding EKG's

Edition V

Dale Dubin, M. D.

Using a modern copying machine, pages 309 to 322 may be reduced or enlarged to fit any personal-reference notebook with a minimum of redundancy in one dimension. Skillful copying of the front and back of each sheet will assure that the information is displayed effectively on both sides of seven sheets. Use a regular sheet of your notebook's paper to mark the holes once the sheets are copied.

May mankind benefit from your knowledge,

Dale Dubin

Dubin's Method
for
Reading EKG's

from: Dubin's *Rapid Interpretation of EKG's*
published by: COVER Publishing Co., P.O. Box 1092, Tampa, FL 33601, USA

1. RATE (pages 61-92)

Say "300, 150, 100" ..."75, 60, 50"

$\frac{1500}{MM} = RATE$

- but for bradycardia:
  rate = Cycles/6 sec. strip × 10

2. RHYTHM (pages 93-189)

Identify the basic rhythm, then scan tracing for abnormal waves, pauses and irregularity.

- Check for: P before each QRS.
  QRS after each P.
- Check: P-R intervals (for AV Blocks).
  QRS interval (for B.B.B.).
- If Axis Deviation, rule out Hemiblock.

3. AXIS (pages 19–228)

- QRS above or below baseline for Axis Quadrant
  (for Normal vs. R. or L. Axis Deviation).
  For Axis in degrees, find isoelectric QRS in a limb lead
  of Axis Quadrant using the "Axis in Degrees" chart.
- Axis rotation in the horizontal plane: (chest leads)
  find "transitional" (isoelectric) QRS.

4. HYPERTROPHY (pages 229-244)

Check V_1 {
P wave for atrial hypertrophy.
R wave for Right Ventricular Hypertrophy
S wave depth in V_1...
+ R wave height in V_5 for Left Ventricular Hypertrophy.

5. INFARCTION (pages 245-288)

Scan all leads for:

- Q waves
- Inverted T waves
- ST segment elevation or depression

Find the location of the pathology (in the L. ventricle), and then identify the occluded coronary artery.

Rate (pages 61 to 92)

from: Dubin's *Rapid Interpretation of EKG's*
published by: COVER Publishing Co., P.O. Box 1092, Tampa, FL 33601, USA

Determine Rate by Observation (pages 74 to 84)

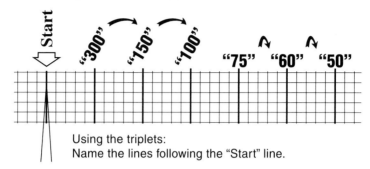

Using the triplets:
Name the lines following the "Start" line.

Fine division/rate association: reference (page 85)

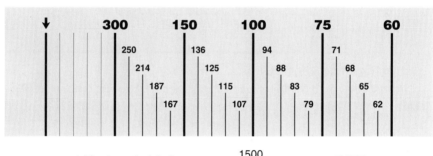

★ May be calculated: $\dfrac{1500}{\text{mm. between similar waves}} = \text{RATE}$

Bradycardia (slow rates) (pages 86 to 92)

- Cycles/6 second strip × 10 = Rate
- When there are 10 large squares between similar waves, the rate is 30/minute.

Sinus Rhythm: origin is the SA Node ("Sinus Node"),
normal sinus rate is 60 to 100/minute

- Rate more than 100/min. = *Sinus Tachycardia* (page 64).
- Rate less than 60/min. = *Sinus Bradycardia* (page 63).

Determine any co-existing, independent (atrial/ventricular) rates:

- Dissociated Rhythms: (pages 149, 152, 175, 176)
  A Sinus Rhythm may co-exist with an independent rhythm from an automaticity focus of another level. Determine rate of each.

Irregular Rhythms: (pages 103-107)

- With Irregular Rhythms (such as Atrial Fibrillation) always note the general (average) ventricular rate (QRS's per 6-sec. strip × 10).

Rhythm (pages 93 to 189)

from: Dubin's *Rapid Interpretation of EKG's*
published by: COVER Publishing Co., P.O. Box 1092, Tampa, FL 33601, USA

★ Identify basic rhythm...

...then scan entire tracing for abnormal waves, pauses, premature beats, and irregularity.

★ Always:

- Check for: P before each QRS.
  QRS after each P.
- Check: PR intervals (for AV Blocks).
  QRS interval (for B.B.B.).
- Has QRS vector shifted outside normal range? (to rule out Hemiblock).

Irregular Rhythms (pages 103 to 107)

Sinus Arrhythmia (page 96)

Irregular rhythm that varies with respiration.

All P waves are identical.

Considered normal.

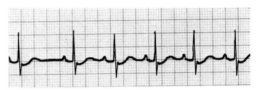

Wandering Pacemaker (page 104)

Irregular rhythm. P waves change shape as pacemaker location varies.

Rate under 100/min....

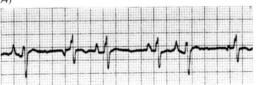

but if the rate exceeds 100/min., then it is called

Multifocal Atrial Tachycardia (page 105)

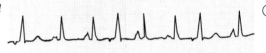

Atrial Fibrillation (pages 106, 159–161)

Irregular ventricular rhythm. Erratic atrial spikes (no P waves) from multiple atrial automaicity foci. Atrial discharges may be difficult to see.

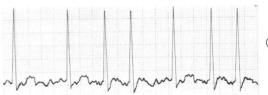

from: Dubin's *Rapid Interpretation of EKG's*
published by: COVER Publishing Co., P.O. Box 1092, Tampa, FL 33601, USA

Escape (pages 108 to 117) – the heart's response to a pause in pacing

- An unhealthy Sinus (SA) Node may fail to emit a pacing stimulus ("Sinus Block"), this pause may evoke an escape beat from an automaticity focus.

pause

(page 115)

Atrial Escape Beat

or

Junctional Escape Beat

(page 116)

or

Ventricular Escape Beat

(page 117)

Then...

the SA Node usually resumes pacing.

- But a sick Sinus (SA) Node may cease pacing ("Sinus Arrest"), causing a automaticity focus to "escape" to assume pacemaker status.

(page 110)

Atrial Escape Rhythm
Rate 60–80/min.

or

Junctional Escape Rhythm

(pages 111–112)

("idiojunctional rhythm")

Rate 40–60/min.

or

Ventricular Escape Rhythm

Rate 20–40/min.

(page 113)

("idioventricular rhythm")

Premature Beats (pages 118 to 140) – from an irritable automaticity focus

- A irritable automaticity focus may suddenly discharge, producing a:

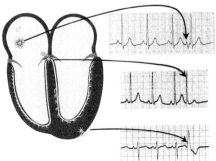

Premature Atrial Beat
(pages 120–126)

Premature Junctional Beat
(pages 127–129)

Premature Ventricular Contraction
(pages 130–139)
P.V.C.'s may be:
multiple, multifocal, in runs, or coupled with normal cycles.

Rhythm continued

from: Dubin's *Rapid Interpretation of EKG's*
published by: COVER Publishing Co., P.O. Box 1092, Tampa, FL 33601, USA

Tachyarrhythmias (pages 141 to 164), "focus" = automaticity focus

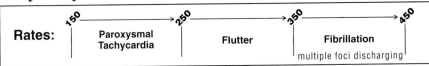

Rates:

150 →	250 →	350 →	450
Paroxysmal Tachycardia	Flutter	Fibrillation	
		multiple foci discharging	

Paroxysmal (sudden) Tachycardia...rate: 150-250/min.

(pages 142 to 153)

"Supraventricular Tachycardia" (page 148)

Paroxysmal Atrial Tachycardia (page 144)

An irritable atrial focus discharging at
150-250/min. produces a normal wave
sequence, if P' waves are visible.

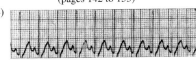

• P.A.T. with block (page 145)

Same as P.A.T. but only every
second (or more) P' wave
produces a QRS.

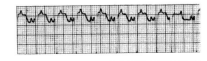

Paroxysmal Junctional Tachycardia

AV Junctional focus produces a rapid
sequence of QRS-T cycles at 150-250/min.
QRS may be slightly widened. (page 146)

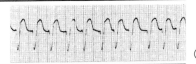

Paroxysmal Ventricular Tachycardia

(pages 149–152)

Ventricular focus produces a rapid
(150-250/min.) sequence of
(P.V.C.-like) wide ventricular
complexes.

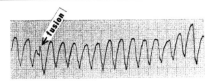

Flutter...rate: 250-350/min.

Atrial Flutter (pages 154, 155)

A continuous ("saw tooth") rapid sequence
of atrial complexes from a single rapid-firing
atrial focus. Many flutter waves needed to
produce a ventricular response.

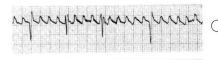

Ventricular Flutter (pages 156, 157) also see "Torsade de Pointes" (pages 153, 231)

A rapid series of smooth sine waves from a
single rapid-firing ventricular focus; usually in
a short burst leading to Ventricular Fibrillation.

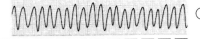

Fibrillation...erratic (multifocal) rapid discharges at 350 to 450/min. (pages 157–163)

Atrial Fibrillation (pages 106, 159-161)

Multiple atrial foci rapidly discharging produces
a jagged baseline of tiny spikes. Ventricular
(QRS) response is irregular.

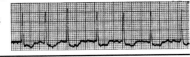

Ventricular Fibrillation (pages 157–163)

Multiple ventricular foci rapidly discharging
produces a totally erratic ventricular rhythm without
identifiable waves. Needs **immediate** treatment.

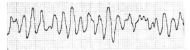

Rhythm continued

from: Dubin's *Rapid Interpretation of EKG's*
published by: COVER Publishing Co., P.O. Box 1092, Tampa, FL 33601, USA

○ **("Heart") Blocks** (pages 165 to 188)

Sinus (SA) Block (page 166) An unhealthy Sinus (SA) Node misses one or more cycles (sinus pause)...

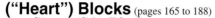

pause

the Sinus Node usually resumes pacing, but the pause may evoke an "escape" response from an automaticity focus.

(pages 115 to 117)

AV Block (pages 168 to 176) blocks that delay or prevent atrial impulses from reaching the ventricles.

Always Check:
- are P-R intervals less than one large square?
- is every P wave followed by a QRS?

1° AV Block ...prolonged P-R interval (pages 168–170). P-R interval is prolonged to greater than .2 sec (one large square).

2° AV Block ...some P waves without QRS response (page 171–174)

Wenckebach: (page 171) ...P-R gradually lengthens with each cycle until the last P wave in the series does not produce a QRS.

Mobitz II: (pages 172–3) ...some P waves don't produce a QRS response. May appear like an occasional dropped QRS.

2:1 AV Block: (page 174) ...may be Mobitz II or Wenckebach. PR length and QRS width help differentiate.

More advanced block may produce a 3:1 (AV) pattern or even higher AV ratio (page 173).

3° ("complete") AV Block ...no P wave produces a QRS response

3° Block: (page 175) P waves—SA Node origin. QRS's—if narrow, and if the ventricular rate is 40 to 60 per min., then origin is a Junctional focus.

3° Block: (page 176) P waves—SA Node origin. QRS's—if PVC-like, and if the ventricular rate is 20 to 40 per min., then origin is a Ventricular focus.

Always Check:
- is QRS within 3 tiny squares?

Bundle Branch Block ...find R,R' in right or left chest leads (pages 177 to 188)

QRS in Right B.B.B. (page 182)   QRS in Left B.B.B. (page 183)

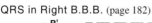

R R'

𝐬 ᴺᵉᵂ
𝕀 + V₆

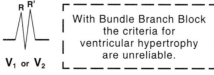

V₁ or V₂

With Bundle Branch Block the criteria for ventricular hypertrophy are unreliable.

R R'

V₅ or V₆

R in I + V₆

Caution: With Left B.B.B. infarction is difficult to determine on EKG.

Always Check:
- has Axis shifted outside Normal range?

"Hemiblock" ...block of Anterior or Posterior fascicle of the Left Bundle Branch (pages 277 to 286).

<u>Anterior Hemiblock</u> (pages 279 to 281)
Axis shifts Leftward → L.A.D.
look for Q_1S_3

<u>Posterior Hemiblock</u> (pages 282, 283)
Axis shifts Rightward → R.A.D.
look for S_1Q_3

Axis (pages 190 to 228)

from: Dubin's *Rapid Interpretation of EKG's*
published by: COVER Publishing Co., P.O. Box 1092, Tampa, FL 33601, USA

General Determination of Electrical Axis (pages 190 to 221)

Is QRS positive (⊥) or negative (⊤) in leads I and AVF?

Is Axis Normal? (page 213)

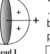

QRS in lead I (pages 202 to 208)
...if the QRS is Positive (mainly above baseline), then the Vector points to positive (patient's left) side.

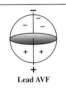
Lead I

Normal: { QRS upright in I and AVF "double thumbs-up sign"

QRS in lead AVF (pages 209–212)
...if the QRS is mainly Positive, then the Vector must point downward to positive half of the sphere.

Lead AVF

First Determine Axis Quadrant
(pages 201– 217)

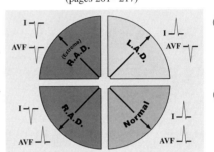

Axis in Degrees (pages 219 to 220) Frontal Plane

After locating Axis Quadrant, find <u>limb</u> lead where QRS is most isoelectric:

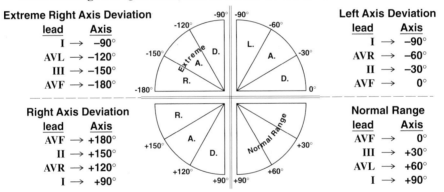

Extreme Right Axis Deviation

lead	Axis
I →	**−90°**
AVL →	**−120°**
III →	**−150°**
AVF →	**−180°**

Left Axis Deviation

lead	Axis
I →	**−90°**
AVR →	**−60°**
II →	**−30°**
AVF →	**0°**

Right Axis Deviation

lead	Axis
AVF →	**+180°**
II →	**+150°**
AVR →	**+120°**
I →	**+90°**

Normal Range

lead	Axis
AVF →	**0°**
III →	**+30°**
AVL →	**+60°**
I →	**+90°**

Axis Rotation (left/right) in the Horizontal Plane (pages 227, 228)

Find transitional (isoelectric) QRS in a <u>chest</u> lead.

transitional QRS
is "isoelectric"

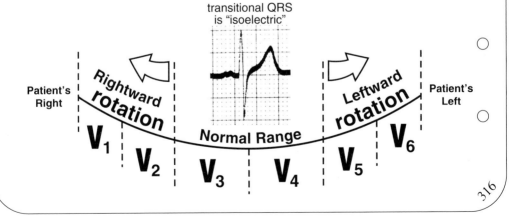

Patient's Right — Rightward rotation

Leftward rotation — Patient's Left

Normal Range

V₁ V₂ V₃ V₄ V₅ V₆

316

Hypertrophy (pages 229 to 244)

from: Dubin's *Rapid Interpretation of EKG's*
published by: COVER Publishing Co., P.O. Box 1092, Tampa, FL 33601, USA

Atrial Hypertrophy (pages 231 to 234)

Right Atrial Hypertrophy (page 234)

- large, diphasic P wave with tall initial component.

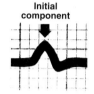

look For
Sharp P in 2

Left Atrial Hypertrophy (page 235)

- large, diphasic P wave with wide terminal component.

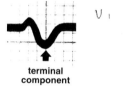

look For
Broad P
in 2

Ventricular Hypertrophy (pages 236 to 244)

Right Ventricular Hypertrophy (pages 236 to 238)

- R wave greater than S in V_1, but R wave gets progressively smaller from V_1 - V_6.
- S wave persists in V_5 and V_6.
- R.A.D. with slightly widened QRS.
- Rightward rotation in the horizontal plane.

Left Ventricular Hypertrophy (pages 239 to 243)

$$\begin{array}{l} \text{S wave in } V_1 \text{ (in mm.)} \\ + \text{ R wave in } V_5 \text{ (in mm.)} \\ \hline \text{Sum in mm. is more than 35 mm. with L.V.H.} \end{array}$$

- L.A.D. with slightly widened QRS.
- Leftward rotation in the horizontal plane.

Inverted T wave:
   slants downward
   gradually,
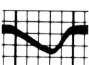
but up rapidly.

Infarction (pages 245 to 288)

from: Dubin's *Rapid Interpretation of EKG's*
published by: COVER Publishing Co., P.O. Box 1092, Tampa, FL 33601, USA

Q wave = **Infarction (significant Q's only)** (pages 257 to 260)

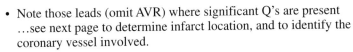
Q

- Significant Q wave is one millimeter (one small square) wide, which is .04 sec. in duration.
  — or is a Q wave 1/3 the amplitude (or more) of the QRS complex.

- Note those leads (omit AVR) where significant Q's are present …see next page to determine infarct location, and to identify the coronary vessel involved.

- Old infarcts: significant Q waves (like infarct damage) remain for a lifetime. To determine if an infarct is acute see below.

ST (segment) elevation = (acute) Injury (pages 252 to 255) **(also Depression)**

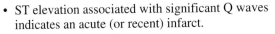
elevation

- Signifies an acute process, ST segment returns to baseline with time.

- ST elevation associated with significant Q waves indicates an acute (or recent) infarct.

- A tiny "non-Q wave infarction" appears as significant ST segment elevation without associated Q's. Locate by identifying leads in which ST elevation occurs (next page).

- ST depression (persistent) may represent "subendocardial infarction," which involves a small, shallow area just beneath the endocardium lining the left ventricle. This is also a variety of "non-Q wave infarction." Locate in the same manner (next page).

T wave inversion = Ischemia (pages 250, 251)

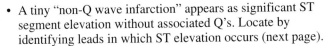
T
inversion

- Inverted T wave (of ischemia) is symmetrical (left half and right half are mirror images). Normally T wave is upright when QRS is upright, and vice versa.

- Usually in the same leads that demonstrate signs of acute infarction (Q waves and ST elevation).

- Isolated (non-infarction) ischemia may also be located by noting those leads where T wave inversion occurs, then identify which coronary vessel is narrowed (next page).

NOTE: Always obtain patient's previous EKG's for comparison!

Infarction Location
— and —
Coronary Vessel Involvement

(pages 261 to 276)

from: Dubin's *Rapid Interpretation of EKG's*
published by: COVER Publishing Co., P.O. Box 1092, Tampa, FL 33601, USA

Coronary Artery Distribution (page 273)

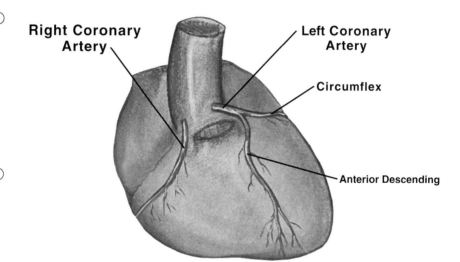

Right Coronary Artery

Left Coronary Artery

Circumflex

Anterior Descending

Infarction Location/Coronary Vessel Involvement (pages 261 to 276)

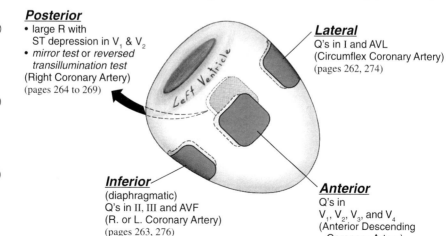

Posterior
- large R with ST depression in V_1 & V_2
- *mirror test* or *reversed transillumination test*
(Right Coronary Artery)
(pages 264 to 269)

Lateral
Q's in I and AVL
(Circumflex Coronary Artery)
(pages 262, 274)

Left Ventricle

Inferior
(diaphragmatic)
Q's in II, III and AVF
(R. or L. Coronary Artery)
(pages 263, 276)

Anterior
Q's in
V_1, V_2, V_3, and V_4
(Anterior Descending Coronary Artery)
(pages 261, 274)

Miscellaneous (pages 289 to 306)

from: Dubin's *Rapid Interpretation of EKG's*
published by: COVER Publishing Co., P.O. Box 1092, Tampa, FL 33601, USA

Pulmonary Embolism (pages 291, 292)

- $S_1Q_3L_3$– wide S in I, large Q, and inverted T in III.
- acute Right B.B.B. (transient, often incomplete)
- R.A.D. and ~~clockwise rotation~~ Counter ? Rish ish wa A Peterson.
- Inverted T waves $V_1 \rightarrow V_4$ and ST depression in II.

Artificial Pacemakers (pages 300 to 304)

Modern artificial pacemakers have sensing capabilities as well as provide a regular pacing stimulus. This electrical stimulus records on EKG as a tiny vertical spike which appears just before the "captured" cardiac response.

Demand Pacemakers: (page 301)

- are "triggered" (activated) when the patient's own rhythm ceases or slows markedly.

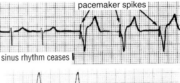

pacemaker spikes

sinus rhythm ceases

- are "inhibited" (cease pacing) if the patient's own rhythm resumes at a reasonable rate.

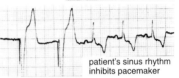

patient's sinus rhythm inhibits pacemaker

- will "reset" pacing (at same rate) to synchronize with a premature beat.

pacemaker ceases at previous timing

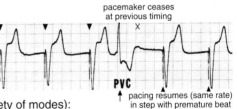

PVC

↑ pacing resumes (same rate) in step with premature beat

Pacemaker Impulse Delivery (variety of modes):

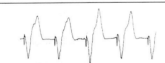

Ventricular Pacemaker (page 303)
(electrode in Right Ventricle)

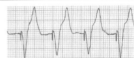

(Asynchronous) Epicardial Pacemaker
Ventricular impulse not linked to atrial activity.

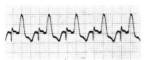

Atrial pacemaker (page 302)

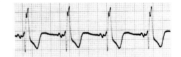

Atrial Synchronous Pacemaker (page 302)
P wave sensed, then after a brief delay, ventricular impulse is delivered.

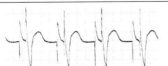

Dual Chamber (AV sequential) Pacemaker
(page 302)

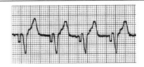

External Non-invasive Pacemaker (page 304)

Miscellaneous continued

from: Dubin's *Rapid Interpretation of EKG's*
published by: COVER Publishing Co., P.O. Box 1092, Tampa, FL 33601, USA

○ Electrolytes

Potassium (pages 293, 294)

Increased K⁺ (page 293)
(hyperkalemia)

+ Narrows

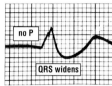

Moderate   Extreme

Decreased K⁺ (pages 294)
(hypokalemia)

Moderate   Extreme

Calcium (page 295)

S+ shortens

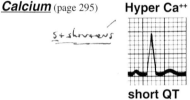

Hyper Ca⁺⁺   Hypo Ca⁺⁺

short QT   prolonged QT

Digitalis (pages 296 to 298)

EKG appearance with digitalis ("digitalis effect")

- remember Salvador Dali.
- T waves depressed or inverted.
- QT interval shortened.

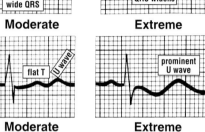

ST gradually slopes below baseline

Digitalis Excess ⟶	Digitalis Toxicity
(blocks)	(irritable foci firing rapidly)
• SA Block	• Atrial Fibrillation
• P.A.T. with Block	• Junctional or Ventricular Tachycardia
• AV Blocks	• multiple P.V.C.'s
• AV Dissociation	• Ventricular Fibrillation

Quinidine (page 299)

Quinidine Effects

- EKG appearance with quinidine (page 299)

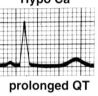

wide QRS

wide, notched P ST depression U wave

wide QT

Excess quinidine or other medications that block potassium channels.
(or low serum potassium)
(page 153)

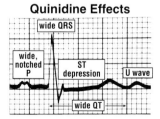

Torsades de Pointes

Practical Tips

from: Dubin's *Rapid Interpretation of EKG's*
published by: COVER Publishing Co., P.O. Box 1092, Tampa, FL 33601, USA

Dubin's Quickie Conversion
—for—
Patient's Weight from Pounds to Kilograms

Patient wt. in kg. = Half of patient's wt. (in lb.) *minus* 1/10 of that value.

Examples:

180 lb. patient	160 lb. patient	140 lb. patient
(becomes 90 *minus* 9)	(becomes 80 *minus* 8)	(becomes 70 *minus* 7)
is 81 kg	is 72 kg	is 63 kg.

Modified Leads
—for—
Cardiac Monitoring

Locations are approximate. Some minor adjustment of electrode positions may be necessary to obtain the best tracing. Identify the specific lead on each strip placed in the patient's record.

Sensor Electrode	Identification	
	Letter	Color (inconsistent)
+	R (or RA)	red
−	L (or LA)	white
Ground (Neutral or Reference)	G (or RL)	variable

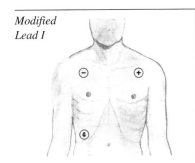

Modified Lead I

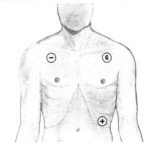

Modified Lead II

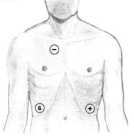

Conventional Lead

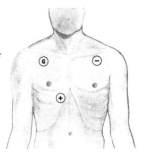

MCl₁
To make this MCl₆ move ⊕ electrode to same (mirror) position on the patient's left side of the sternum.

EKG Tracings

This section contains EKG tracings (and their interpretation) from various patients. The tracings and interpretations are provided so that you can see how this method of reading EKG's actually works. Try these few examples so that you grow accustomed to this systematic approach. Once you learn how to read an EKG systematically, you will soon become very skilled at routine EKG interpretations.

Patient D.D. is a 29 year old white male known to be a hypochondriac with numerous complaints.

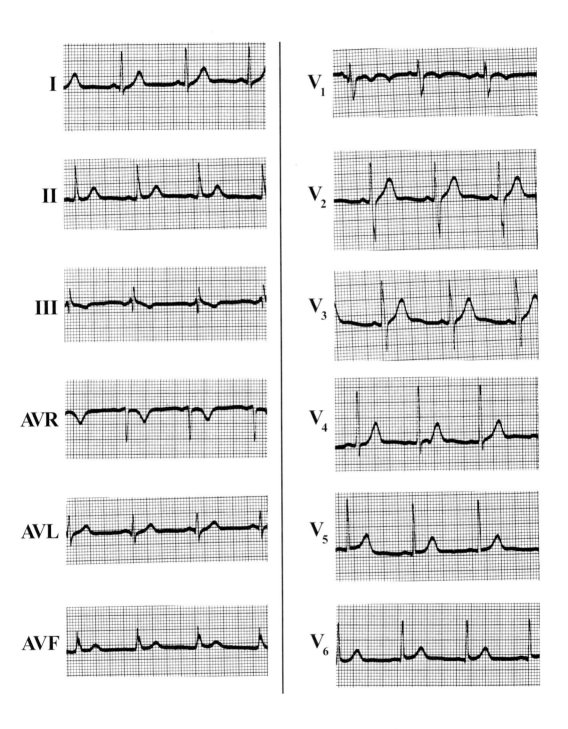

EKG Interpretation

Patient: D.D.

Rate: about 70/minute

Rhythm: Regular Sinus Rhythm
P-R less than .2 sec. (No AV Block).
QRS less than .12 sec. (No B.B.B.).
     …but note the R,R' in III suggesting incomplete
     Bundle Branch Block.

Axis: Normal Range (about +30°).
Rightward rotation in the horizontal plane.

Hypertrophy: No atrial hypertrophy.
No ventricular hypertrophy.

Infarction: No significant *Q waves.*
(coronary
vascular
status)
                ST segments—not elevated, except for V_5 and V_6 where ST
     is elevated 1/2 mm. due to "early repolarization."*
T waves—generally upright.

Comment: This is an essentially normal tracing. This is the author's
own EKG, however he is no longer 29 years old.

---

* Early repolarization is characterized by (minimal) ST elevation in the left chest leads, often with counter-clockwise rotation (horizontal plane). It is a normal finding in young athletic males.

Patient R.C. is a 45 year old black male with a history of coronary vascular disease. Blood pressure was 210/100 on admission.

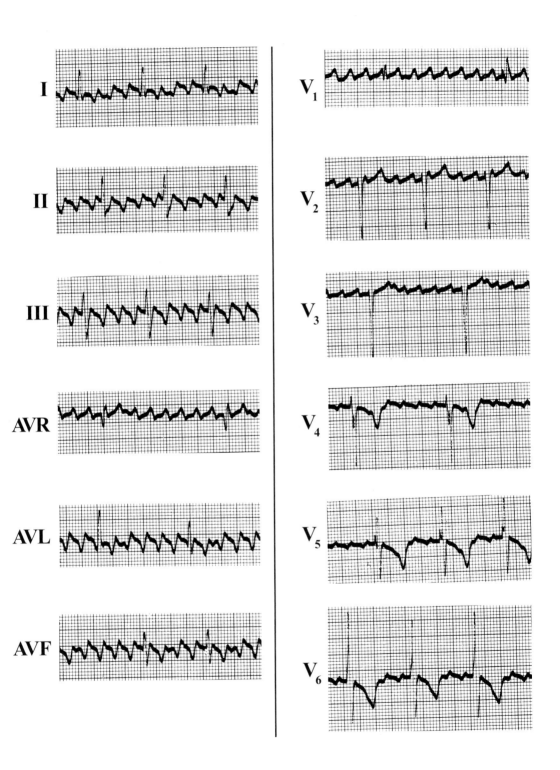

EKG Interpretation

Patient: R.C.

Rate: Atrial rate of 300/minute
              Ventricular rate generally 60/min. but occasionally slower.

Rhythm: Atrial Flutter (with inconsistent ventricular response, i.e.,
                no fixed AV ratio).
              P-R is variable.
              QRS is less than .12 sec. (No B.B.B.).

Axis: Left Axis Deviation (-30°).
              Leftward rotation in the horizontal plane.

Hypertrophy: Atrial hypertrophy difficult to determine.
              No ventricular hypertrophy.

Infarction: *Q waves*—Q in lead I (also note large S in Lead III).
(coronary   *ST segments* are generally isoelectric.
vascular   *T waves* are inverted in I and AVL (look closely)
status)   and the mid-to-left chest leads.

Comment: The most obvious problem is Atrial Flutter with an atrial rate of 300/
              min. and a variable irregular ventricular rate (average circa 60) caused
              by the variable AV conduction ratio between 3:1 and 7:1. An old occlu-
              sion of the Left Circumflex Coronary artery is evidenced by the old
              lateral infarction. New involvement of the Anterior Descending Coro-
              nary artery is suggested by anterior ischemia (T wave inversion in V_4,
              V_5, V_6), as well as by the probable Anterior Hemiblock (shift to Left
              Axis Deviation with Q_1S_3 configuration; previously R.A.D. with his
              old lateral M.I.). Note that if one scrutinizes the T wave regions (some-
              what obscured by flutter waves) in the limb leads, the flutter waves dip
              lower (suggestive of negative T waves) rather than higher (if superim-
              posed on upright T waves) in all but AVR, indicating a generalized
              cardiac ischemia, as well as the obvious compromise of both branches
              of the Left coronary Artery.

Patient K.T. is a 61 year old obese, black male who was brought into the emergency department by his family. This patient had a sudden episode of severe left chest pain. Blood pressure was 95/65.

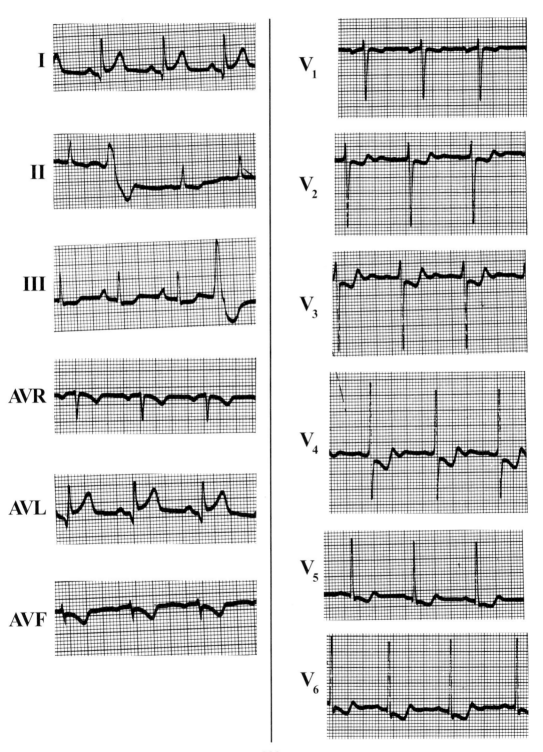

EKG Interpretation

Patient:	K.T.
Rate:	about 75/minute
Rhythm:	Generally regular Sinus Rhythm with occasional P.V.C.'s. *P-R* is exactly .2 sec. so we will have to say there is a borderline first degree AV Block. *QRS* is less than .12 sec. (No B.B.B.).
Axis:	Left Axis Deviation (nearly -90°). No rotation in the horizontal plane.
Hypertrophy:	Probable left atrial hypertrophy. Left ventricular hypertrophy.
Infarction: (coronary vascular status)	*Significant Q waves* in I and AVL. *ST segments* are elevated in I and AVL. ST segments are depressed in V_1, V_2, V_3, and V_4. *T waves* are flat or inverted in II, III, and AVF and all chest leads.

Comment: This patient has a classical acute lateral infarction caused by an occlusion of the Left Circumflex Coronary Artery. Coincident with this is a probable occlusion of the Right Coronary Artery characterized by prominent R waves with ST depression in the (V_1 to V_4) chest leads. Also, T wave inversion in II, III, and AVF suggests Right Coronary compromise. T wave inversion in all chest leads is indicative of ischemia of the Anterior Descending Coronary Artery. Note also the tall, peaked T waves in I and AVL known as "hyperacute T waves," which, although uncommon, characterize a very acute M.I. The Left Axis Deviation appeared in this patient's previous EKG's and is most likely related to his left ventricular hypertrophy rather than implicating Anterior Hemiblock (also, the Bundle Branch System appears to conduct normally). Occasional P.V.C.'s caused by the ischemia, depending on frequency and multiplicity of origin, may forebode more serious arrhythmias.

Patient G.G. is a 45 year old Asian male who was doing heavy work when he was overcome by severe, crushing, anterior chest pain. Blood pressure was 110/40 on admission to the hospital.

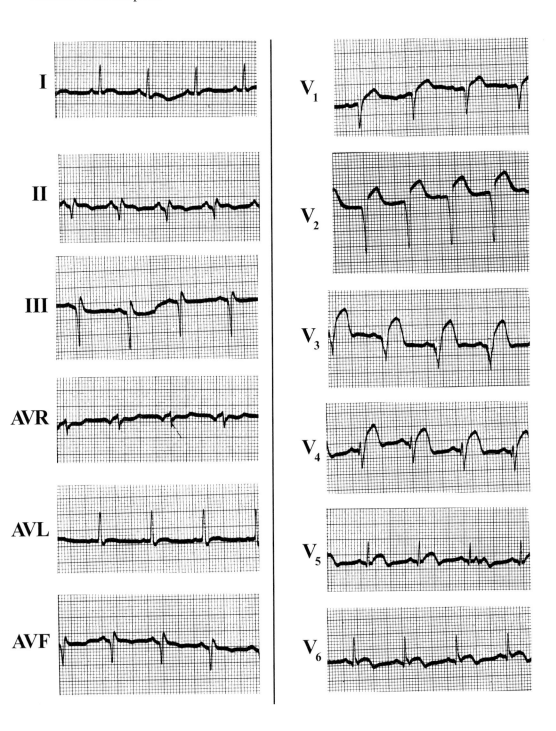

EKG Interpretation

Patient: G.G.

Rate: about 100/minute but variable.

Rhythm: *Sinus* Rhythm, somewhat irregular due to Sinus Arrhythmia.
              P-R less than .2 sec. (No AV Block).
              QRS less than .12 sec. (No B.B.B.).

Axis: Left Axis Deviation (-30° to -60°).
              Leftward rotation in the horizontal plane.

Hypertrophy: No atrial hypertrophy.
              No ventricular hypertrophy.

Infarction: *Significant Q waves* in II, III, and AVF.
(coronary   There are also very large Q waves in V_1, V_2, V_3, and V_4.
vascular   *ST segments* are elevated in V_1, V_2, V_3, and V_4.
status)   *T waves* are difficult to distinguish, but inverted T waves
              are noted in V_4, V_5, and V_6.

Comment: This patient has an acute antero-septal infarction, probably representing an occlusion of the Anterior Descending branch of the Left Coronary. Generalized ischemia of the myocardium is evident by the flat-
to-inverted T waves in nearly every lead. The old inferior infarction
demonstrated on this EKG was noted on the patient's previous hospital
record and is the documented etiology of his Left Axis Deviation (no
Hemiblock). Note that the QRS becomes isoelectric between V_4 and V_5
but this is *not* within the normal (V_3, V_4) range; this represents minimal
leftward rotation away from the septal infarction. Old EKG's showed
no anterior involvement on his previous admission.

Patient E.M. is a 65 year old hispanic female. She was admitted to the hospital because of constant left chest pain for twelve hours. Blood pressure on admission was 110/75.

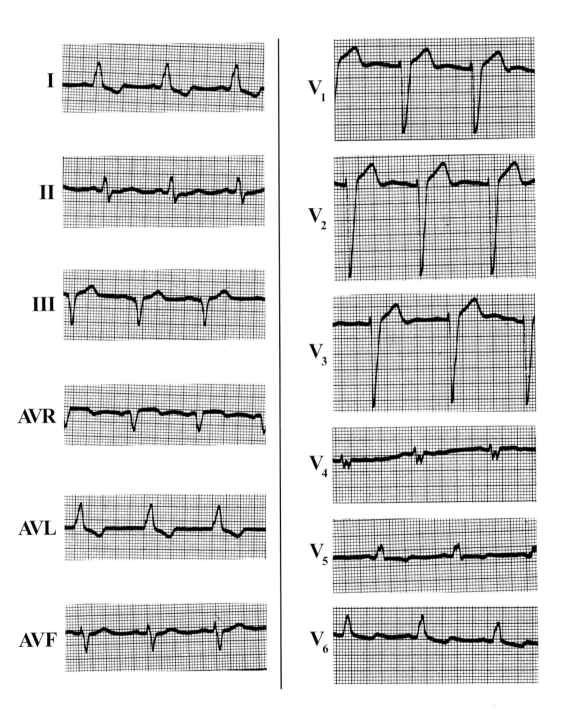

EKG Interpretation

Patient: E.M.

Rate: 60/minute

Rhythm: Sinus Bradycardia
P-R is about .2 sec. so there is probably a
  first degree AV Block.
QRS is more than .12 sec. (it is .16 sec. wide). R,R' is present in
  V_5 and V_6 so there is a Left Bundle Branch Block.

Axis: Suggestive of Left Axis Deviation, but not reliable because of the
  presence of Bundle Branch Block.

Hypertrophy: No atrial hypertrophy.
Ventricular hypertrophy is difficult to determine
  because of Bundle Branch Block.

Infarction: *Q Waves*—not a reliable criterion of infarction in the presence of
(coronary   Left Bundle Branch Block.
vascular   *ST segments*—not reliable in the presence of Left Bundle
status)   Branch Block.
T Waves are flat in V_4, V_5, and V_6, but not reliable with
  Left Bundle Branch Block.

Comment: Enzyme studies confirmed a presumptive diagnosis of myocardial
infarction. The patient's chest pain made us suspicious.

Patient M.A. is a 75 year old black female with a long history of marked hypertension.

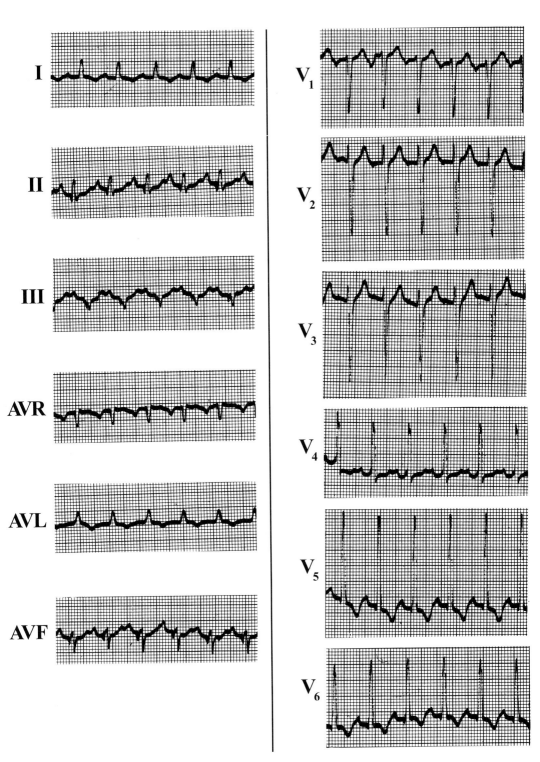

EKG Interpretation

Patient:	M.A.
Rate:	about 125/minute
Rhythm:	Sinus Tachycardia *P-R* is less than .2 sec. (No AV Block). *QRS* is less than .12 sec. (No B.B.B.).
Axis:	Left Axis Deviation (minimal amplitude of QRS in limb leads make exact axis determination difficult). No rotation in the horizontal plane.
Hypertrophy:	Left atrial hypertrophy. Left ventricular hypertrophy with strain.
Infarction: (coronary vascular status)	*Q waves* are present in II, III, and AVF. *ST segments*—generally isoelectric (on baseline), but V_5 and V_6 show strain pattern. *T waves* are inverted in I and AVL, and also in V_5, V_6.
Comment:	This patient has hypertrophy of both the left atrium and left ventricle with a left ventricular strain pattern. The patient also had an old inferior infarction. The Left Axis Deviation is caused by the Mean QRS Vector pointing away from the (old) inferior M.I. and toward the thickened left ventricle. It does *not* represent Hemiblock. There is currently (lateral) ischemia in the distribution of the Left Circumflex Coronary Artery.

R.M., an anxious, obese, 57 year old white male whose law practice was failing, complained of "tight, squeezing" pain in his anterior chest. An electrocardiogram was quickly taken by an Emergency Medical Technician.

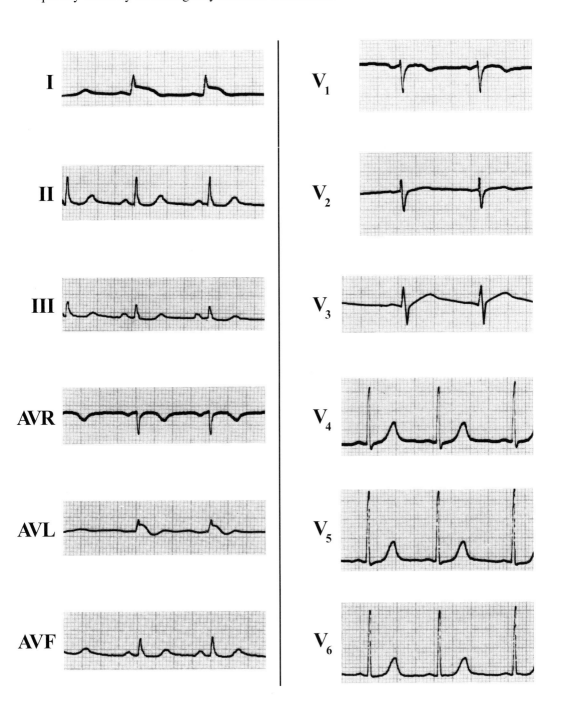

EKG Interpretation

Patient: R.M.

Rate: 75/minute

Rhythm: Sinus Rhythm
P-R .16 sec. (No AV Block).
QRS .08 sec. (No B.B.B.).

Axis: about +45° (Normal).
No rotation in the horizontal plane.

Hypertrophy: Possible minimal left atrial hypertrophy.
No ventricular hypertrophy.

Infarction: *Q waves*—no significant Q waves.
(coronary vascular status)   *ST segments*—elevated 2+ mm. in I and AVL.
T waves—inverted in I and AVL.

Comment: It is interesting that in this innocuous appearing EKG there is a subtle non-Q wave infarction in the lateral left ventricle, which very soon developed into a serious lateral infarction. Symptomatology suggestive of M.I. always must be investigated and scrutinized.

Index

Index

Index

Index

Index

Thunderbird, 44-45
Time measurement, 33, 34
Torsades de Pointes, 153, 294, 299
Transplant, heart, 305
 heterotopic, 306
Trifascicular Block, 286
Trigeminy, ventricular, 135
Triplets, 76-80
Twelve Lead EKG, 52

Vagas Nerve, 57, 59
Vaso-vagal syncope, 57, 59
Valve:
 aortic valve, 18
 AV Valves, 15-16, 20
   Mitral valve, 16, 18,
   Tricuspid valve, 16-17
 pulmonary valve, 17
Vector, 190-227
 determination, 201-228
 deviation (in frontal plane), 207-208, 214,
                       238-239
 locating, 201-217, 228
 normal, 213
 rotation (in horizontal plane), 222-228,
                       238-239
 with Infarction, 199-200, 228
 with Ventricular Hypertrophy, 198, 200, 228
Ventricle, 197, 283
 Left, 7, 18, 239-243, 247-248
 Right, 7, 17, 237-238, 273, 275
Ventricular Conduction System, 20-21, 98
Vertical heart, 197, 283
Voltage, 31
Vulnerable period, 139

Wandering Pacemaker, 104, 107
Waves
 delta, 189
 flutter, 154
 P, 14-15, 19, 29
   diphasic, 233
   flat, 293, 299
 P', 104-105, 107, 110, 114, 119, 121-123,
         144-147, 231, 286
   inverted P' (retrograde) 112, 128
 q (insignificant), 23, 257-258
 Q, 23, 185, 257, 259-260, 291
 QS, 25
 R, 24, 75, 240-241
 S, 24-25, 82, 241, 291
 T, 26-29, 139
   flat, 294
   hyperacute, 328-329

T wave, continued
 inverted, 250, 291-292
   asymmetrical, 242
   symmetrical, 251
 peaked, 293
 U, 98, 294, 299
Wenckebach, 171, 174
White, P.D., 189, 288
Wilson, F.N., 48
Wolff-Parkinson-White (Syndrome), 189

342

AFIB

lone
Paroxysmal —converts itself
Persistent
Permanent

low voltage

Pericarditis (effusion, tamponade
hypothyroid
COPD

Inverted T on a Q (Prolonged)
MAY be seen
in
3, AVR and OR V₁

---

if Early transitions c CP
R/o MI c 2A echo
Posterior wall MI